Relating Experience
Stories from Health and Social Care

Edited by Caroline Malone, Liz Forbat,
Martin Robb and Janet Seden

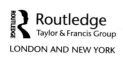

Routledge
Taylor & Francis Group

LONDON AND NEW YORK

TheOpen
University

First published 2005
by Routledge
2 Park Square, Milton Park, Abingdon, Oxon OX14 4RN

Simultaneously published in the USA and Canada
by Routledge
270 Madison Ave, New York, NY 10016

Routledge is an imprint of the Taylor & Francis Group

© Compilation, original and editorial matter, The Open University 2005

Typeset in 10/12 Sabon by Wearset Ltd, Boldon, Tyne and Wear
Printed and bound in Great Britain by TJ International Ltd, Padstow,
Cornwall

British Library Cataloguing in Publication Data
A catalogue record for this book is available from the British Library

Library of Congress Cataloging in Publication Data
A catalog record for this book has been requested

ISBN 0-415-32657-5 (hbk)
ISBN 0-415-32658-3 (pbk)

CONTENTS

INTRODUCTION

Martin Robb and Liz Forbat

It is often said that interpersonal communication and relationships are at the 'heart' of health and social care. Communicating effectively and developing productive relationships, whether between care providers and service users or within organisations, are increasingly seen as central to the process of improving the quality of care services. A great deal of media and public attention has been focused in recent years on apparent failures or breakdowns in communication, whether between care professionals and the public or between different agencies. As a consequence, a range of initiatives have been designed to improve communication skills and processes, and to transform the nature and quality of relationships in care services. The emphasis is increasingly on openness, participation and partnership, even if the reality of everyday experience in care settings does not always live up to these high ideals.

Central to developing better communication and relationships is improving understanding of what is involved in these diverse and complex processes. A key part of this is gaining an awareness of how service users, carers and care professionals actually experience their everyday interactions. Listening to the voices of those involved at all levels in health and social care, as they recount their experience and reflect on the meanings it has for them, is essential. Engaging with firsthand accounts of personal experience, while not a substitute for academic analysis, can work alongside it in a complementary way, providing powerful examples of what makes for both 'good' and 'difficult' encounters in the context of care, illustrations of the changing nature of caring and professional relationships, and insights into how communication and relationships might be improved.

There is an increasing recognition of the value and importance of narrative and biographical accounts, as well as of creative and imaginative responses to experience, in both research and practice in the care sector. Stories of whatever kind, and whether of 'real' or 'imagined' experience, can give a sense of the texture of experience and provide insights that may be absent from conventional academic and policy texts. This does not mean assuming that all (and only) experiential accounts provide an 'authentic' insight into everyday realities in care settings. Rather it involves an acceptance that even the most 'objective' accounts are themselves constructed as narratives, and that it is only by attending to a range of different 'stories' that we can build up a picture of the diversity and complexity of encounters and relationships.

This anthology provides a diverse selection of accounts of interpersonal communication and relationships in the context of health and social care. By far the majority of the items included are personal accounts of direct experience by people using or working in care services. Most are contemporary and many have been written especially for this anthology. However, the book also includes other kinds of accounts, including attempts to encapsulate in fictional, poetic and visual form something of the nature of encounters in the context of care. Although this is not primarily an academic volume, there is also a sprinkling of more analytical accounts that are intended to complement and support the more experiential material.

Each of the extracts illustrates the importance of different kinds of communication when building and sustaining relationships in health and social care settings. The extracts were chosen because each of them, in different ways, reflects on how relationships are created and sustained and their impact on satisfaction whether for service users or practitioners. They indicate the ways in which both practitioners and service users can begin to critically evaluate their own interactions within these settings: thinking about what works well, what assumptions are embedded in such encounters, and what they would like to happen differently if faced with a similar situation in the future. The accounts reflect a wide diversity of viewpoints and include the voices of service users and providers, as well as those who have experience of both roles. They include personal experiences located *within* health and social care contexts as well as reflections *on* these locations as organisations. Although attempts have been made to encompass a diversity of viewpoints, no selection of this length can be exhaustive or entirely representative. The power of the extracts reproduced here lies in their capacity to enable readers to take a fresh and critical look at their own experience, and to use that experience to re-evaluate their own understanding of interpersonal communication and relationships in the context of care.

USING THE BOOK

This anthology has been designed to be used by a variety of readers, for a diversity of purposes. Both users of health and social care services and those who work in them will find material here that will enable them to reflect on their own experience of encounters and relationships. Students on a wide range of courses in health and social care will want to use the extracts reproduced in the book as case material to support their study of interpersonal communication, and the organisation of the book into separate sections should help them to select relevant readings. The book is also a set text for the Open University course Communication and Relationships in Health and Social Care (K205), which aims to encourage those involved in health care, social work and social care to reflect critically on their everyday interactions and relationships and to develop their practice. This book is intended as a companion volume to the course Reader (Robb *et al.*, 2004). The course materials refer to this anthology at regular intervals and course activities invite students to reflect on and analyse the extracts included here. However, the book also includes additional items not referred to directly in the course, and readers are encouraged to browse through the book and follow up links suggested by the introductions to each part.

The anthology is divided into five parts, each of which has a distinctive focus. The introduction to each part provides an overview of its contents, drawing attention to links between items and to relevant material elsewhere in the book. Deciding on topics for the five parts – on changing relationships; the way things happen; the physical context of care; difficult encounters; and working together – was not an easy task. There are also a number of cross-cutting themes, such as power, and difference and diversity along the axes of gender, ethnicity, age and class.

Part I takes the reader on a journey through time, with the accounts included here illustrating changes in the nature of relationships in the context of care and also changes in the way those relationships have been understood. The extracts in *Part II* explore different aspects of the process of communicating and relating in care settings, covering ways of helping, good and not-so-good experiences, and pointing to skills which can enable people to improve their interactions. *Part III* focuses on the physical and situated nature of communication. These extracts span the life-course and offer commentary on a range of physical differences, from specific illnesses and impairments to reflections on the environment in which health and social care is delivered. *Part IV* explores particularly 'difficult' encounters from a range of different perspectives. While each of the accounts presents a harrowing experience, the authors work hard to reflect on how communication in each of these instances impacted on different layers of relationships. Finally, *Part V* looks at the part played by communication in 'working together', whether in groups and teams or more widely across institutional boundaries.

This anthology has been assembled by the editors from suggestions made by members of the K205 course team at The Open University. Besides the four editors, other course team members involved in the selection and discussion of material for the book have been Sheila Barrett, Ann Brechin, Jenny Douglas, Linda Finlay, Anne Fletcher, Carol Komaromy and Anita Rogers. Secretarial support was provided by Val O'Connor, the course team assistant. Finally, thanks are due both to those who contributed original material for the anthology and those who gave permission for their work to be reproduced from elsewhere.

REFERENCE

Robb, M., Barrett, S., Komaromy, C. and Rogers, A. (2004) *Communication, Relationships and Care: a Reader*, London: Routledge/The Open University.

PART I

CHANGING RELATIONSHIPS

INTRODUCTION

Martin Robb

The extracts in this first part of the book illustrate some of the ways in which relationships between providers of care and those they care for, as well as between people working in health and social care services, have changed over time, as well as highlighting some important continuities. Included here are autobiographical accounts, extracts from imaginative literature, and more academic attempts to theorise the changing nature of relationships in the context of care.

The opening poem by the 16th-century writer John Owen demonstrates that there is little that is new in the ambivalence with which care professionals are regarded. The group of readings that follows recount personal stories that illustrate relationships in care settings in the more recent past. Ranging from the time of the First World War to the 1990s, these accounts demonstrate the apparent persistence of paternalism and deference, but also a slow but inexorable shift in attitudes and expectations.

The account by American Catholic social activist Dorothy Day, of her 'war work' as a nurse in 1918, evokes the almost military hierarchy that existed in hospitals at the time, while at the same time illustrating the acts of kindness and consideration that were possible in this often harsh context. Alan Bennett's account of his parents' contact with doctors provides a vivid illustration of how the medical profession was regarded in a northern working-class community in the 1940s, immediately before the advent of the National Health Service. Doctors were lofty and distant figures, belonging to a different social class to most of their patients. Much more intimate was the relationship with the local 'wise woman': it was only when her ministrations failed that doctors were resorted to. The recollection of medical training in a London teaching hospital in the 1960s by Ghada Karmi, a Palestinian refugee, shows just how embedded were relationships of paternalism and deference. In Karmi's account, consultants and senior medical staff treat both junior doctors and patients with haughty disdain, while the latter respond with either passive acceptance or scarcely concealed fear.

In 'Birth memories' the anonymous author remembers her experience of giving birth in hospital in the mid-1970s. With one exception, she recalls the midwives' treatment as authoritarian and prescriptive with little room for personal autonomy. By contrast, when she herself trained as a midwife in the 1980s, the balance of 'kindness and cruelty' had shifted. 'Training as a mental nurse in the 1960s' conjures up a harsh and paternalistic world where medical staff knew what was best for patients and, despite the kinds of reservations expressed by the author, subjected them to treatments such as ECT against their will, on the pretext that it was in their interests.

The anonymous account of 'Changes in social work relationships' tells a complex story of changing public perceptions of social workers, and the ways in which these in turn have shaped relationships with clients. Easygoing relationships are shown as being replaced by fear in the aftermath of anxieties about child abuse, but then becoming more supportive again as policy and practice changed. It is a powerful example of how political and ideological changes can impact on the nature and quality of both caring and professional relationships. 'Communication and Caribbean transnational families', while it does not deal directly with relationships in care settings, has been included to illustrate both how the experience of migration affects relationships and also the ways in which changing communication methods impact on those relationships, often in unexpected ways.

Theodore Dalrymple's article provides a link between these recollections of past

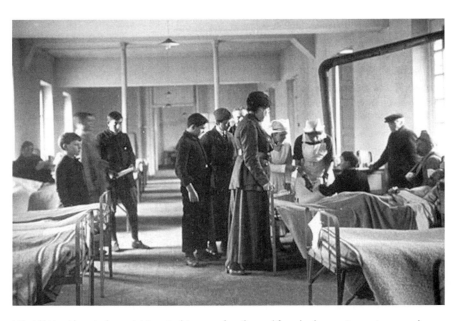

World War I hospital ward. Historical image of uniformed female doctors (centre) on ward rounds at an American Women's Hospital, France. (Source: Stanley B. Burns MD and The Burns Archive, NY/Science Photo Library)

experience, and the more analytical reflections that follow. Drawing on his experience as a doctor, the author argues that there has been a widespread (and in his opinion regrettable) shift in British people's expectations and practice of interpersonal communication. According to Dalrymple, the emotional reticence of the older generation has been replaced by a pervasive emphasis on emotional expression (what he terms 'emotional incontinence') at all costs.

Sami Timimi's account of how changing theoretical perspectives have led him to rethink his own practice as a child psychiatrist is perhaps more measured. Both experiential and analytical, this piece is a demonstration of the power of ideas to shape and to transform practice. Among the ideas that have influenced 'post-modern' practitioners like Timimi have been those of the French philosopher Michel Foucault, whose work is the focus of the final extract by Madan Sarup. Though more explicitly theoretical than many of the items in this anthology, this piece has been included because it is part of a wider story about changes in ways of thinking about caring relationships. Coming at the end of the section, it throws retrospective light on the reasons behind some of the changes and continuities exemplified by the preceding accounts.

ONE

'GOD AND THE DOCTOR'

John Owen (c.1563–1622)

God and the Doctor we alike adore
But only when in danger, not before;
The danger o'er, both are alike requited,
God is forgotten, and the Doctor slighted.

Source: *The Oxford Dictionary of Quotations*. Oxford: Oxford University Press, 1999.
Reproduced by permission.

TWO

KING'S COUNTY

Dorothy Day

From the beginning I enjoyed the work. In 1918 nursing was a simpler thing than it is today. We went on the ward at seven in the morning and our work day lasted twelve hours. For two hours in the afternoon we were off duty, not to rest, but to attend lectures on materia medica physiology or anatomy. For the first three months we were probationers and wore pink uniforms with big white aprons. At the end of three months we passed to blue and white striped dresses with stiff white collars and a white starched cap, of which we were most proud. For three years until graduation this was the uniform, and then we wore white.

There was strict etiquette. You stood when a head nurse entered the ward. You stood aside for your seniors to pass through a door first. You were taught an almost military deference and respect for the superior officer, or for the doctor. From the first, in addition to bed-making and care of the ward, we were given nursing to do, straight nursing, which delights every woman's heart. We had to keep charts, but there was a minimum of paper work. We took temperatures and pulses, gave medicine, baths, alcohol rubs, distributed trays, gave hypodermics, enemas and douches. We tried to make the patients comfortable, and changed sheets daily. Never have I seen such a profligate use of bed linens, eggnogs and medicines as during that year at King's County Hospital. My experience there reassured me as to the care one received from the city. It was a care given to citizens, not to paupers. And it was all free. Of course, we had nothing to do with the social service department so saw nothing of the interviewing of the poor.

My first patient was an old Canadian woman, ninety-four years old. Granny objected to being bathed, saying that she had bathed the day

Source: Day, D. *The Long Loneliness*. San Francisco (CA): HarperCollins, 1952/1980.
Reproduced by permission.

before and at her time of life she did not see why she had to be pestered with soap and water the way she was. Argument was useless, so she began to fight with the nurses, clawing at them and screaming and sitting in the middle of her bed like a whimpering monkey.

'Let us help you,' one of the other nurses said soothingly. 'Can't you see that we want to take care of you, because we love you?'

'Love be damned,' the little old lady cried, 'I want my wig.' And she began to cry and whimper again. She sat there perched on the end of her thin spine, her eyes blazing black and clear. Her arms were clasped about her bare and scrawny knees. Around a large bare spot on her head she had a thin fringe of hair which stood up like a field of ferns.

'She has been crying for her wig since she came in,' the other nurse said. 'We let her have her teeth, but she wants her wig. I don't see why they don't let her have it.'

It was Miss Adams who was my companion in the work. She was Catholic and stood out at once in my mind. [. . .]

She had sympathy and understanding and realized that the little old lady needed more than soap and water and clean bed linen. She needed more than to be loved. She wanted to be respected as a person, and for that she needed to have her wishes respected. She needed such appurtenances as her wig. I remember we compromised with a cap and so pleased her.

There were two women dying in the ward, a woman of fifty and a girl of twenty-two. Mary Windsor was slowly fading from the whiteness of the ward around her into a gray shadow on the long slim bed. She had a grown son who came to visit her every evening when the wards were twilit and the evening toilets were completed. He brought bunches of flowers which were fragrant and colourful, and every time I passed the bed, a thrill shook me, life and death were so close there. Mrs. Windsor never spoke but lay motionless, looking out of wide gray eyes, looking at the death she saw so plainly, with a dull wonder.

Irma was pathetically young. Her finely shaped mouth was always con-torted with pain and there was a fierce protesting light in her eyes. The lines that agony had drawn in the ivory skin were like those of passion. She might have been clutching a lover in a last embrace, knowing that when he rose from the bed he would go out and close the door forever. There was the smell of death around her, I kept thinking, and there was no one to bring her flowers to deaden it.

For a while I worked on the fracture ward where there were old ladies with fractures of the hip and leg. The most youthful of them were over sixty years. They approached the elderly stage when they were eighty and when they had passed ninety-five it was admitted they were old. It seemed strange at first to call them by their Christian names, but it was the custom of the hospital and I soon became used to it.

This ward broke me, the work was so hard. There was one bearded woman with no breasts and the nurses spoke of her furtively as being a freak. She was ugly in temper, threw things at the nurses, and was filthy in her habits so that she constantly needed to be cleaned. She tried to spit at the nurses and to dirty their clean uniforms. It was an ugly trial to care for her. I had to grit my teeth and hold my breath while I washed her, to control my aversion.

Working on this ward was the hardest part of my hospital career. One afternoon when I had been cleaning up filth all day, and the perverse patient had again thrown her bedpan out on the floor dirtying my shoes and stockings, I left the ward in tears and sat in the washroom weeping uncontrollably at the ugliness and misery of life. I could not stop crying long enough to tell Miss Adams, so that my patients would not be left alone, but did the unforgivable thing and ran away, going to my room where I continued to cry. I shall always remember with what gentleness the assistant superintendent of nurses came and talked to me about the responsibilities of the nurse and the dignity of her profession and the 'sacrament of duty.' She might not have used those words, but that was the tenor of her talk and I have never forgotten it. She took me off the dif-ficult ward for the time, transferring me to medical where there were fifty patients with influenza. This was the time of the 'flu' epidemic and the wards were filled and the halls too. Many of the nurses became ill and we were very short-handed. Every night before going off duty there were bodies to be wrapped in sheets and wheeled away to the morgue. When we came on duty in the morning, the night nurse was performing the same grim task.

For a time I was on the men's medical ward and Miss Adams and I were alone all day from seven until seven, excepting time for meals. We were so short-handed that the head nurse had to take the ward on the floor above and could only occasionally run down to advise us.

There was one head nurse, a Swede, who was a martinet. She used to come and look over our wards with a grimly critical eye, watching for care-lessness, for unevenness in the lining up of the beds, for a spread awry, for a cluttered bedside table. It was hard not be careless at this time when every day ten or twelve new patients were carried in or walked staggeringly only to fall unconscious as soon as their clothes were taken from them.

According to this nurse, each ward in the hospital should be in order by ten o'clock every morning. In order to get the work under way Miss Adams and I went without our breakfasts in the nurses' dining room and came on the ward at six-thirty. There we could take a hasty cup of coffee and count on a mid-morning snack after the dreaded visit of the head nurse was over. There were a few up-patients who helped us and without them we would have had a harder time. I remember Red Reynolds, who had been a bartender in Coney Island, and who now was in charge of the diet kitchen. He used to give us scrambled eggs, toast and coffee every morning and helped us make eggnogs for the patients on the ward.

When we went on duty in the morning, the up-patients were already at work, sweeping, polishing, getting the linen in order and helping other weaker patients into their wheel chairs. These were trundled out into the solarium, where they sat all day, chewing tobacco and gossiping of wine, women and war and occasionally of God. Sometimes you could hear the cracked voice of a sailor singing a chanty or the booming voice of an old German whose bones were turning to stone singing a hymn.

My first task was to pour out the medicine for a hundred patients, a task demanding concentration and a steady hand. When I first started pouring, I continued it in my dreams every night until I was able to associate every patient with the medicine which he took. For instance whenever I saw Smith, my brain immediately flashed

Arom. Spt. Am. Dr. 1
Donov. Sol. M. 10
Pot. Iod. Gr. 15
Stokes M. Dr. 1

There were almost as many mixtures for each patient, and it was a job which took two hours.

Nursing was like newspaper work. It was impossible to suffer long over the tragedies which took place every day. One was too close to them to have perspective. They happened too continuously. They weighed on you, gave you a still and subdued feeling, but the very fact that you were continually busy left you no time to brood.

There was a brightness of the sun pouring in on the ward and over the white spreads and the feeling of spring in the air. Out in the grounds on warm days the patients from the old people's homes sat together, men and women, and it was tragic to think that some of them were married and could not spend their last days together. They smoked, many of the women, and had their pipes and tobacco just like men, but in that year it was still a rare thing for a woman to be seen smoking a cigarette and the nurses were not permitted to smoke. I used to snatch a surreptitious smoke by taking a roundabout walk behind the powerhouse and laundries going to and from the nurses' home. What discipline I submitted to because I loved the work!

THREE

PROPER NAMES

Alan Bennett

My parents' names are Lilian and Walter, Lil and Walt as they call each other. Except that they don't very often, particularly after my brother and I are born, which somehow puts paid to their names. When we come along, Walter and Lilian are buried and thereafter they are almost always called Mam and Dad, not merely by us, but by each other, their names deferring to their function as parents.

Occasionally, though, function forgotten, they resume their identities and become people again and it is always at times of pain or stress. As when, sometime in the early forties, Mam has the last of her teeth out. Dad has had all of his taken out at one go when he is twenty-five, but Mam loses hers more slowly, until one of her front teeth having decayed so spectacularly it looks as if it may snap off, she has all of hers out too.

After this wholesale extraction she is in terrible pain. Someone tells her that cigarettes help and we come home from school to find her crouched over the fire inexpertly puffing at one of Dad's cigs (the first and only time in her life that she smokes), her legs, as women's were in those days, mottled red and black from sitting too close to the fire. When Dad comes home, he isn't Dad but Walt and she is Lil, holding his hand and weeping by the fire with a vinegar and brown paper plaster stuck to her aching face.

The next time Mam is Lil is just after the war when Dad, who is unemployed and has been ill on and off for six months, collapses one Sunday morning in the street in Armley and, having managed to reach the house of a friend, he lies on the floor crying out with excruciating pain.

He is a patient of Dr Moneys who has hitherto dismissed his symptoms as 'wind', prescribing what Dad calls 'another bottle of that chalky muck' and which my brother or I are sent down the road to fetch from Timothy

Source: Bennett, A. *Telling Tales*. London: BBC Worldwide Ltd, 2000. Reproduced by permission.

White's the chemists. The chalky muck doesn't do the trick and whatever it is that has felled Dad to the kitchen floor, it plainly isn't wind.

Dramatic though the circumstances are, a doctor is not lightly to be called out on a Sunday morning, though how readily a doctor does 'come out', particularly at night or out of hours, is what makes him, irrespective of his diagnostic skills, a good doctor, and certainly a good doctor to be with – 'He'll always come out,' the highest praise a patient can bestow.

This is 1946, on the eve of the introduction of the National Health Service, and the Armley doctors Dr Gordon and Dr Dalrymple are still rather lofty figures, living in some style, or in detached houses anyway with brass plates on the gateposts, and on this Sunday morning probably up at Adel playing golf.

Even in poorer Wortley where we are currently living with Grandma, the doctors are quite grand, Dr Moneys and Dr Slaney, distinguished silver-haired figures exercising a paternal sway over their slum practices, not poor particularly or seemingly over-worked, and still with all the old-fashioned accoutrements of their profession – the pin-stripe suit, the watch chain and the Humber parked in the empty street – so that any visit by the doctor is noted by neighbours in those otherwise careless days.

But before it's decided to get a doctor or an ambulance, someone runs up the street to knock on the door of a woman who knows a bit about medicine and minor ailments to see if she can gauge the urgency of the situation. Someone else must have run up to the Whingate terminus to get a tram down to Wortley to fetch my mother, whose name Dad is now calling, and that it is 'Lil' he is calling, not 'Mam', diagnosis enough that whatever the woman up the street may say, he, at least, thinks he is dying.

That there is a wise woman on hand is not unusual, as such figures are a customary part of working-class life and provide an unofficial auxiliary medical service. In those days, though, the remedies they purveyed and their dabbling in matters medical at all were more officially disparaged, any resort to them to be kept quiet when seeing 'the proper doctor'.

There is no shortage of such folk doctors. The street in which Dad has collapsed is in the Moorfields, and this group of streets is home to such a woman. We had once lived half a mile away in the Hallidays and there is one there too, a Miss Thompson. She is someone to whom Dad goes with minor complaints and generally boils, a boil particularly on the back of the neck a more regular affliction than it is now, the square of lint and the sticking plaster with which it is covered making the sufferer walk in a way both stiff-necked and wary, thus imparting to their gait a vaguely Vorticist slant. Miss Thompson generally blames the blood and prescribes burdock root, which is bought at a herbalist in one of the back streets near Leeds Market where herbs jostle with trusses and remedies for piles and more complicated and mysterious surgical appliances that make it a shaming place for a child to visit – or a child like me, anyway.

Originating in such a marginal emporium the burdock, at any rate in my mother's eyes, retains a taint of the truss and so has to be prepared in a strictly circumscribed fashion, steeped in a special basin before being boiled up in a chipped blue enamel pan, uniquely designated for the purpose as 'the herb pan', and never to be used for the sprouts, say, or the potatoes; Dad dosing himself with the resultant liquid over a longish period generally without bothering to decant it from the pan, a practice my mother predictably deplores.

Besides the blood, wise women like Miss Thompson are apt understandably to lay the blame for the body's ailments on the bowels, so when today the wise woman comes down the street, still wiping her hands on her apron from doing the Sunday dinner, she takes one look at Dad and blames constipation and for this she has the remedy to hand. Dr Moneys, at his most airily detached, could not have got it more wrong or embarked on a procedure more calculated to give excruciating pain and broadcast the infection throughout the gut, because what Dad is suffering from, screaming out with now, is a perforated ulcer and what she is suggesting is an enema.

Perhaps she brings her own enema, though in any case there would be one in the house, as there certainly is in ours.

Coiled black and serpentine in its almost new box, with the instructions pasted underneath the lid, the enema looks like a section of the innards it is meant to irrigate, the hard liquorice-coloured bulb at the same time suggesting some ancient musical instrument. I feel it must have been precaution more than necessity because ours has never been used; otherwise no amount of washing would manage to cleanse it, and it would certainly not be in the sideboard drawer as, in Mam's eyes, use would have polluted it for all eternity and it would have been consigned to the murky cupboard below the bathroom basin or stowed with other permanently tainted articles in the ghetto behind the cistern.

By the time my brother and I arrive in our caps and gabardine raincoats, never other than neat even in the presence of death – or what we think is death – it is to find Dad, his torture just having been administered, laid out on the floor of this strange kitchen, with Mam holding his hand as he gives vent to the terrible cries of her name.

'Lil.' 'Lil.' 'Lil.' And it is the name as much as anything that tells us this must be death.

Now the ambulance arrives and he is taken to St James's – these days known nationwide as Jimmy's from its numerous TV appearances. It isn't then – St James's is just a poor alternative to the Infirmary. Both, though, are old hospitals, Gothic and even picturesque, and it's in one of the wards, now I think a museum, where Dad is admitted to be operated on that night, my brother and I kneeling down by our attic beds to pray for him like children in a Victorian painting.

For almost a week he is critical and nowadays would, I suppose, have been kept in Intensive Care. Each patient has a number, printed every night in the *Yorkshire Evening Post*, Dad's often in the dreaded category, 'Friends may visit', the words unprinted being 'before it's too late'. He catches pneumonia, as patients tend to do, and for a time is moved into the bed by the door, the significance of which I only learn years later at the Old Vic when watching Peter Nichols' play *The National Health*, the bed by the door generally taken to be the anteroom to the mortuary.

But it isn't, and eventually Dad pulls round, is brought home to Grandma's at Gilpin Place where a bed is made up in the sitting room, and he lies in state, waiting eagerly for my brother and me to come home from school every afternoon when he can ask us what we've been doing, something that he has never done before, maybe because he hasn't had the opportunity, but which makes me think, almost for the first time, that perhaps he actually likes me.

But now things are back to normal, Lil and Walt banished again; he is Dad and she is Mam, their names put back in the drawer to be kept for best – or worst. Or perhaps, too, for those times when I wake in the night and hear them in bed, talking and laughing, being themselves.

FOUR

MEDICAL TRAINING IN THE EARLY 1960s

Ghada Karmi

The early months of 1963 were bitterly cold. There were prolonged snow-falls that year and we were glad that we would spend the worst of the weather in lodgings in Southmead Hospital. Our consultant teachers varied; a few were gentle, but the majority were capricious egoists. It was on the 'firms' – study groups of ten or so students – that we were closely subjected to their paternalism and their arbitrary exercise of power over us. Anxiously, we studied their every vagary because the medical world operated on a system of networks and personal recommendations and it was important not to offend. Everyone dreaded the fate of the mythical houseman (junior hospital doctor) who, having completed his first house job (as pre-registration hospital appointments were known) received a reference from his consultant to this effect: 'Dr So-and-so tells me that he has been my houseman for the last six months.' Or, in a variation of the story, the reference went: 'This man has been working for me over the last six months to his own satisfaction.' The reign of fright we lived under merely reinforced for me the paternalism and prohibitions of my childhood.

Nor were the patients any more protected from these medical prima donnas than we were. On one of the medical firms, I remember that we came into contact with the senior chest physician, a Dr Pearson. He was a dapper, well-dressed man who had the air of an aristocratic younger son. His speciality brought him into contact with a large population of patients, mostly men with chronic bronchitis. They were inexplicably devoted to him, for he treated them all like old family retainers, never addressed them

Source: Karmi, G. *In Search of Fatima. A Palestinian story*. London: Verso, 2002.
Reproduced by permission.

by anything except their surnames and was remarkably unsympathetic to their plight. If patients, wheezing and coughing, and so short of breath they could scarcely walk, ever complained of their condition, he would say briskly, 'No use complaining, Smith,' – or Jones or Wilson – 'you're living on borrowed time, hmm? Realise that, do you?'

And they would answer, 'Thank you very much, sir, thank you.' One day, while taking us on one of his ward rounds, he stopped by the bed of a patient with a collapsed lung. The patient's chest had been fitted with a tube, connected to a positive pressure appliance which helped him to breathe. The tube ran down the side of the bed and, as Dr Pearson stood beside the patient explaining the case to us, he leant unthinkingly against it. His weight shut off the tube and the patient, who was already having difficulty breathing, started to protest feebly. But Dr Pearson, looking towards us and unaware of the problem, mistook this for another of the complaints he usually dismissed.

'Quiet, Dickson, there's a good chap. Lucky to be alive, hmm?' But the man's distress increased and when his face turned blue we could no longer stay silent. 'Sir,' said one of us timidly, for consultants were never to be interrupted or corrected, 'Sir, I think the patient's tube is shut off.' At this, Dr Pearson started and, looking down at the constricted tube, jumped away smartly from the bed and called the nurses. As the patient was revived, he patted him over the head and said, 'Terribly sorry, old thing. Didn't mean to. Better now?' And, to our surprise, the man nodded with no hint of reproach.

FIVE

BIRTH MEMORIES

Anonymous

Many vivid memories from giving birth in the mid-1970s have stayed with me. Over time I seem to have distilled those of the midwives who cared for me into two main categories. There were midwives who were extremely kind and those who were not. Sadly, the former were in the minority. One sister glows in my memory as the embodiment of calmness and kindness. The interesting thing is I cannot remember any specific words that she said to me. When finally I went into labour, I begged her to deliver my baby, and she apologised and smiled and made a reassuring comment about her colleague looking after me just as well. Instead, her colleague told me to 'stop making that noise!'

The midwife who admitted me two nights previously was not kind and it is interesting that I remember many of her words. Here is a selection. She laughed at me: 'What do you mean you don't know if your waters have broken?' She frightened me: 'You will *know* when you go into labour!' And, the next night, she threatened me: 'If you haven't had that baby by the time I come back tonight *I'll* get it out of you!'

The threat and Syntocinon seemed to work and I went into labour the next lunchtime. Debbie was born at 2pm after a rapid delivery, but I didn't see her until 2 o'clock the next day. Apparently I needed my rest. Anything less conducive to rest is difficult to imagine.

Thereafter, I was not allowed to have my baby with me at night but, because of the amount of milk I was producing, a concession was made for me to visit the nursery once, to feed Debbie, but for no longer than 45 minutes. There were many other strange restrictions on my personal liberty. For some reason I have yet to understand, I was not allowed to wash my hair.

When I was discharged (at eight days instead of ten and 'don't say we didn't warn you if you bleed') I was told by a senior midwifery sister, 'Don't forget, normal babies sleep for 20 out of 24 hours.'

My baby was definitely not normal!

As a midwife in the 1980s, I discovered that the balance of kindness and cruelty had shifted. Most midwives really enjoyed being 'with women', just like the sister who glows in my memory.

SIX

TRAINING AS A MENTAL NURSE IN THE 1960s

Anonymous

In the late 1960s, between the ages of 18 and 21 years, I trained in a large mental hospital, which housed 1200 inmates, to become a Registered Mental Nurse. At first I thought that all of the patients were mad and dangerous and the staff were sane and normal. As l learned more about the subtleties of mental illness, the boundaries between psychiatric diagnoses became increasingly blurred and between 'us' and 'them' less tenable. But the relationship between theory and practice remained divided.

On the wards things were different. Staff, and in particular psychiatrists, knew better than their patients did what was good for them. This seemed reasonable for those who had committed terrible crimes and were in locked wards and on powerful drugs, later called chemical straitjackets. But for those patients who were depressed and for whom there was no easy relief through medication, the only treatment on offer was ECT (electro-convulsive therapy), and this seemed unreasonable. In the hospital, twice a week, up to 100 patients were given ECT.

When I worked on the female admission ward up to 21 patients were treated twice a week with ECT and it was part of my role to persuade patients to consent to this treatment. If they did not, then we had the power to treat them against their will, but for 'their own good'. I dreaded having to coerce patients into modified ECT treatment and occasionally help to drag people into the dormitory. I was relieved when patients co-operated or walked into the dormitory often in a zombie-like state.

Although we thought that we knew better than the patients did what was good for them, no one understood how or why ECT worked – if it did. There were many theories about why a current being passed through someone's brain and producing an epileptic-like fit should relieve depression, but it was all speculative.

I hated what I did and am still embarrassed and ashamed. Perhaps the worst thing, apart from the danger and cruelty, was the relationships of trust that were destroyed. Each week I had to look into the face of someone who did not want be treated and manage the hypocrisy of pretending that it was in her interest.

SEVEN

CHANGES IN SOCIAL WORK RELATIONSHIPS

Anonymous

In the early 1970s I trained as a generic (general) social worker and worked in hospitals, children's departments (as they were then) and also in the probation service, which meant visiting prisons as well as working with people in the community. I recall working with many troubled, disadvantaged and supposedly dangerous people during that time. I remember feeling safe most of the time, and experienced a degree of acceptance from the clients I worked with which I found surprising and had not expected.

There were set procedures for the work, but I also found that I had a great deal of personal choice and autonomy about the way I worked with the people allocated to me in the 1970s. For example, I could choose to take children to see a parent in prison. I could work with families until they chose for the work to end. I could argue about the injustice of women being arrested for soliciting when kerb crawlers were not arrested (as they can be now) with management and get agreement not to take them back to court. I could argue for parole for prisoners on the grounds of their children's suffering from the sentence. It was also true that callers to the children's department or to the probation office were rarely turned away. If someone said they needed help with either a child or a probation-related matter, the usual thing was to offer whatever assistance you could within the agency's means. I was usually free to offer that to clients on request in addition to the allocated work I had.

There was great emphasis on building relationships with clients and communities and responding to demand. Relationships with other workers were largely informal and it was common practice to phone other agencies and ask for their help over the phone for callers and actually get it – there and then. Professional 'wisdom' and 'authority' were seldom questioned by clients or other agencies in a way that I found quite scary and persistence usually paid off when seeking resources from other agencies for clients. I felt that on the whole I could respond to what service users were asking me to do to quite a significant degree and create some change. By the late 1970s there seemed to be more resources and the benefits system seemed more flexible too, so that advising people on entitlements was very productive.

In 1977 I took a career break to be with my three small children and returned to work half-time in the new social services department in 1984. Social workers were still able to work with all groups, older people, people with mental health issues, children and families but most specialised to some degree. I chose to work mainly with children and family issues. While I had been away child care practice had changed and the resources available to help families had become much more stretched. During this time Social Security Benefits were much reduced and many of the one-off grants (e.g. for moving house, children's clothing) had been cut. This left social workers with less practical assistance to offer, as before helping people to make the most of the benefits system was a real possibility for improving their opportunities.

The work seemed to me driven by rules and procedural manuals and only prioritised families were offered any help. Families would comment 'I suppose I have to bash my kids to get any help from you lot.' This was true, as most of the allocated work was with families where a child had been thought to be injured or neglected by a parent. There was also an emphasis on supervising and checking. There was little place for family support work and you were not encouraged to accept requests for advice and guidance from parents who were 'not on the register'. There was much more paperwork and meetings, many of which were formal and meant families had to come to the office. Visits were much more routine and planned with agendas set more by workers and less by the service users. There was no time for community activities.

Further, I was amazed by the changes to people's perceptions of social work. When I knocked on doors I wasn't as welcome as before. Gone was the idea of a 'friendly authority' person. In its place was the idea of the nosy, busybody, interfering social worker who went around checking up on people. I began to enjoy the work with older people more, who still seemed to think I was there to help. For a while this change was a barrier to my practice with families. I learned gradually to work with this new perception of my role and tried to work with the hostility and to understand how it was created by the way the child care system had become investigative and stretched for resources.

I found it helped to be honest about the way the role had changed and how service users felt about it. People no longer wanted to be associated with the stigma of having a child care worker calling. They did however expect the best from the service and were much more openly critical and assertive, a good thing except when it became threatening and abusive. Most people would concede 'you're only doing your job, someone has to.' However, I did feel that often the approach was narrow and prevented families from working to and identifying their own strengths. Also I felt that the agency would hold a case conference on a family to 'be on the safe side' when really some simple support and advice would have reduced the family's stress and built up their confidence as parents. Being 'conferenced' could be a negative and deskilling experience. Working to involve families and make the experience positive felt like an uphill struggle against 'watch your back' styles of management. It also meant families would hide things from you. I was relieved to find when I asked several of the families I visited if there was a reason why they had just got big fierce dogs that they said it was to see off the city council rent arrears bailiffs, not me!

Relationships with colleagues had also become more formal. There were regular meetings of all the people who worked in the geographical area. Notes were made and partnership plans agreed. Discussions of joint approaches to individual families were a feature of practice and I was much more aware of working as part of a team of practitioners with agreed plans and had less sense of personal autonomy and choice. This was often supportive and helpful and protected service users from practitioners' whims but it also raised some complicated issues about 'what you said to whom' and 'who said what when' and the whole idea of client confidentiality was more complicated. Managers took a much more proactive role too in making sure that a team approach to families was consistent with departmental policies about the allocation of resources. Managers from each agency would meet and devise shared policies and procedures. Often this meant resources were shared more fairly but sometimes it turned into simple cost cutting.

Later, I was able to work in a children and family centre and manage a range of support services. This was great for me because, while I still had to work carefully to child protection procedures and account for resources, I was able to work with people who came to the centre looking for support as well as those who were 'sent' by professionals. The centre offered a range of therapeutic groups, training on parenting skills and the needs of children, sessions on play and child behaviour as well as individual support sessions and practical help. Parents were on the management group and had a real say in the programme and activities. Parents could also set up their own groups and networks. The relationships with parents were very relaxed and it was possible to know the children well, and meet their needs in a detailed way. It was also possible to offer coffee to parents and to sit in the lounge to talk over their worries and difficulties. Often referral to the social service protection team was needed, but it could be talked over and agreed.

In 1989 the Children Act produced a swing back to an emphasis on working in partnership with parents and meeting children's needs as well as safeguarding them from harm. This coincided with my move to university teaching, but it has begun to make an impact in the 1990s and early 2000s. On reflection, swings in policy and the way these are interpreted make a big difference to the relationships between service users and workers and between workers. It is to be hoped that the philosophies of the Children Act will enable practitioners to get something of a balance, although alas the image of the social worker seems to be permanently damaged by the rigour of 1980s practice and the media attention to supposed failures. There is a lot of good work out there that just does not get reported!

EIGHT

COMMUNICATION AND CARIBBEAN TRANSNATIONAL FAMILIES

Anonymous

Communication is a particular concern for many minority ethnic communities living in the UK. Many individuals migrated from the Caribbean, Indian subcontinent and Africa in the 1950s and 1960s for economic reasons, planning initially to stay in the UK for relatively short periods of time and then return to their country of birth. Some families, disillusioned with prospects in the UK in the 1970s and their experiences of racism, migrated again to North America – Canada and the USA. More recently, some people from the Caribbean have returned to their country of birth on retirement or have retired to North America.

In my case, my parents were born in Jamaica and migrated to England in the 1950s: my father first, followed by my mother. I was born in Wolverhampton as part of a large extended family of aunts, uncles and cousins who had also migrated to England. By the 1960s many of my relatives were becoming disillusioned with the realities of life in the UK. In fact my own parents planned to return to Jamaica but stayed in the UK because they believed in the benefits of the British education system. Many of my aunts and uncles migrated again to Canada and the USA.

My husband migrated from Barbados in the 1960s. His mother left Barbados initially leaving her three children to be cared for by her sister, who had no children of her own. This was quite commonplace during migration. Once my husband's mother was settled economically in England, and now with a new family, he and his sisters joined her. It must also be remembered that, before the migration from the Caribbean to the UK in the 1950s, there had been a history of migration within the Caribbean and to the USA and Canada. Thus migration and the processes associated with it has been a central part of family life in the Caribbean during the 20th century. Such family connections spread across continents are part of everyday life for many people from the Caribbean and increasingly so for many other communities where people choose to migrate to other countries for a variety of reasons.

Goulbourne and Chamberlain in their research on transnational Caribbean families say:

> *While it could be expected that family links over time would weaken, as distance, ageing and death reduced the emotional ties and the material obligations, our research indicates that on the contrary those direct family links have continued through the generations, and have been strengthened by return migration and by easier and cheaper communications. Indeed the 'revolution' in communications has changed the shape of migration itself.*
>
> Goulbourne and Chamberlain, 2001, p. 41

These writers point to the increased availability of cheap flights, and contend that many individuals can return to their country of birth, or countries where they have lived, with greater frequency and can 'replenish cultural contacts'.

For me, this has been particularly true. With close family in Florida, Toronto, Barbados and Jamaica, the decreased costs of international telephone calls and flights and the greater access to email and the internet have not only maintained close family ties but also have developed an international awareness and perspective in our children. Many of my older relatives have become computer literate so that they can communicate with relatives by email.

Recently my husband's father died in Barbados. The death of a close family member is always stressful and is compounded by distance. However, being able to talk with other family members by telephone is now more accessible for many people. The nature of communication changes when you cannot see people face to face and must discuss feelings and worries by telephone without being guided by the usual non-verbal cues. It possibly means that there is a greater reliance on verbal communication and listening and being prepared both to express how you feel and to enquire how the other person feels more directly. Migratory processes have meant that we have no relatives living close to us and so I could not attend my father-in-law's funeral as I needed to be with our children. However, because of ease of access to a telephone, my husband and I were able to stay in touch throughout his stay in Barbados and give each other support. In some ways we possibly talked more about the death than we might have done had we not been separated by distance.

REFERENCE

Goulbourne, H. and Chamberlain, M. (2001) *Caribbean Families in Britain and the Trans-Atlantic World*, London, Macmillan Education Ltd.

NINE

THEY'VE GOT TO GET IT OUT OF THEIR SYSTEMS

Theodore Dalrymple

The first thing that strikes me about Britain whenever I return home from abroad is the lack of dignity of the people, and their complete absence of self-respect. Almost the entire population looks as though it has let itself go: and considers itself right to have done so. It is militantly slovenly.

Poverty has nothing to do with a lack of self-respect. Long residence and extensive travel in Africa have taught me that extreme poverty and a precarious existence are not incompatible with a fierce self-respect. Nor was the British population always like this. My mother, a refugee to this country more than 60 years ago, tells me that the first thing she noticed about the British – of all classes – was their quiet dignity. Now the first thing she notices as she steps out of her door is the shamelessness of their public conduct.

The sudden change has been wrought in part by a gestalt switch in our attitude towards the public expression of emotion. Where once emotional restraint and self-control were admired, now it is emotional incontinence that we aim for. It is as if we had undergone potty-training in reverse.

The British have been thoroughly persuaded that emotions are like pus in an abscess. If they are not released – by screaming and shouting, hugging and crying, wailing and raging, and the more publicly the better – they will turn inwards and cause a kind of emotional septicaemia. The person who controls himself is not only a figure of fun, but a traitor to his own best interests.

The signs of this collective loss of control are everywhere, and have made the British – in my view quite rightly – despised around the world, at

Source: Dalrymple, T. *New Statesman*, 16–30 Dec 2002. Reproduced by permission.

least everywhere they congregate in any numbers. It is only natural that those who believe that self-control is wrong should also think that social disinhibition is good: in effect, that the worse they behave, the better they are.

A newspaper once sent me to observe the behaviour of the English football fans at a match abroad. The man behind me, who had a good job, spent hours shouting obscene abuse and making quasi-fascist gestures (in unison with thousands of others) at the team and supporters of the home country. During one brief interlude of comparative silence, I asked him why he had come all this way to behave like this.

'I've got to get it out of my system,' he replied.

'Why have you got to?' I asked. I received no reply. Far from being cathartic, is it not more likely that in the public expression of obscenity, as in other kinds of conduct, practice makes perfect?

The mass public drunkenness that is to be seen at least three nights a week in the centres of all British cities and towns, for example, is one natural consequence of the idea that to control yourself is harmful, and has something distinctly ideological about it: for it is the ultimate triumph of the doctrine of disinhibition as mental and social health. Yet the yells and screams, the raucous laughter and querulousness that invariably accompany this drunkenness are not, to my ear at least, the sound of spontaneous gaiety, but rather of hysterical desperation.

The idea that the public expression of emotion is always and everywhere a good thing has several baleful consequences. It debases our culture by the loss of subtlety, by making our culture so crude and literal-minded; and at the same time it fosters the grossest insincerity while reducing people's ability to detect it. (I used to be amazed that millions of Americans were unable to see at a glance, from the very first moment that they appeared on the screens, that televangelists were charlatans at best and outright crooks at worst. But now, it seems to me that the British have become thoroughly susceptible to the same crudity of manipulation.) The logic of the doctrine leads to an incessant inflation of modes of expression: and he is deemed to feel most who most successfully draws attention to himself.

It is significant that advertisements which seek to portray happiness or fun now increasingly show people screaming with laughter, their huge mouths cavernously open, as if people were no longer able to interpret any lesser indications of pleasure. The result is histrionics on a mass scale, as each person tries to make his emotion obvious to others.

It is possible for suppression of emotion to go too far. I see this very often, for example, among older Indian women who are my patients, and who are deeply unhappy with their domestic circumstances. Unable, for social and cultural reasons, to confess to this unhappiness, and likewise, for the same reasons, unable either to leave the home or sublimate their unhappiness by other forms without physical pathology as an expression of their misery. Their symptoms last for years or even for decades, and they are dragged round to doctor after doctor by their complicit relations in an attempt to reach a diagnosis that will never be reached.

But the emotional restraint of the British for which they were known not so very long ago, is still present in the older generation, and to me comes as a great relief, almost balm to my soul, whenever I meet it. Contrary to what is often supposed, it was not a class phenomenon, but a general cultural one that extended across society (if anything, the upper classes had less of it); and it gave to people precisely the dignity of which my mother spoke.

Not long ago in the corridor of my hospital, I met the husband of a patient of mine. He was in his early seventies, and was deeply jaundiced. At that age, the most likely diagnosis was secondaries in the liver. I greeted him and remarked that he didn't look very well.

'I'm not feeling very well,' he said, 'but I'm going for tests.'

About two weeks later I met him again.

'It's not very good news, I'm afraid,' he said – by which, of course, he meant he would be dead soon.

'I'm sorry to hear that,' I said.

'We'll just have to make the best of it we can,' he said, and I wished him well.

In a few simple words, he conveyed nearness to death: and I expressed my sympathy for him, which he understood to be genuine precisely because it was undemonstrative and proportionate to the sorrow a comparative stranger might properly be expected to feel for another, without the need to fake anything. I didn't claim to be devastated, that I should never recover, or even that I wouldn't be able to eat my dinner that night with enjoyment: no I meant what I said, which was that I was sorry to hear it.

What moved me about the exchange was that, by not letting himself go in front of me, he, only a few weeks before his death (in fact he died two weeks later), tried to avoid embarrassing me. Even as he faced death, a social obligation was important to him. I can only hope, when my turn comes, I meet it with such dignity.

This fortitude was a cultural characteristic and great virtue of the British, now utterly smashed up by the doctrine of self-expression. I am thinking of what one old working-class lady, who had suffered real tragedy throughout her life, told me when I asked her whether she ever cried. 'Indoors,' she replied. 'But not when I'm out. It wouldn't be right, would it, doctor, to burden others with my troubles?'

While an emphasis on emotional expressiveness is inherently self-regarding, appropriate to a nation of egotists, emotional restraint is an inherently social, or other-regarding, quality. In my view, it is vastly more attractive, and far from deadening people emotionally, it sensitises them to nuances that grosser forms of expression extinguish altogether. Emotional incontinence, moreover, encourages self-importance and self-absorption: a process that is all too visible in our media. Our horizons become limited, out sympathies involuted. The world is of less importance to us than the trivial fluctuations of our emotional state. Self-pity becomes the dominant factor of our lives and destroys all perspective.

It also destroys a sense of humour. An ironical detachment from one's own woes – once so marked a characteristic of the British, and indeed their finest characteristic – becomes impossible, and is replaced by a perpetual querulous sense of grievance. Why am I not happy all the time? It is my right to be happy all the time. Therefore, someone must be depriving me of my entitlement.

The difference between the old and the young of these islands is not one merely of age, such as there has always been. I don't think that the emotionally incontinent young, who believe that public displays of feeling are the *sine qua non* of an emotional life, will one day mature into stoics. They have been too thoroughly indoctrinated in the supposed virtues of emotional expressiveness for that. Their own old age will be terrible; and their cultural tastes are destined to remain crude and unrefined. The constituency for restraint in both art and life will grow even smaller.

TEN

THE NEW PRACTITIONER: THE EMERGENCE OF THE POST-MODERN CLINICIAN

Sami Timimi

After completing my general psychiatric training, I decided that I wanted to pursue a career in child and adolescent psychiatry. Already I had realised that I could not pursue a career in adult psychiatry where, as far as I could see, the dominance of biopsychiatry meant becoming a glorified pharmacist, dispensing medication.

My training in child and adolescent psychiatry proved no less confusing, however. I went from prescribing medication on no more than a handful of occasions to prescribing for every patient, outpatients and inpatients. I went from making grandiose interpretations that focused on the complex emotions between family members, to ignoring all emotions and focusing only on the behaviour of an individual child. And I went from focusing on early mother–infant history, to focusing exclusively on here and now forward-looking approaches.

I began to realise that in mental health circles, professionals are not so much in the job of discovering the reason behind a client's difficulties; rather, they are often more interested in creating a set of meanings to explain them. In other words, as mental health professionals we make new stories out of the stories that patients tell us.

But where were the connections, the cross-over points, the integration? Maybe I was too sensitive to difference. Perhaps I should have been more accepting and, like a well-behaved trainee, learned to live with all this. After all, living with ambivalence was one thing that my cultural upbringing had taught me (I lived in Iraq until the age of 14, when I moved to England).

Source: Timimi, S. *Young Minds Magazine*, vol. 62, Jan/Feb 2003. Reproduced by permission.

IDENTITY PROBLEM

But I began to realise also that child psychiatrists have a real identity problem. We are, after all, doctors by training. And within child and adolescent mental health services, we are at the top of the hierarchy – in positions of influence and power and, usually, the most highly paid professionals. Yet there are few drug types available for us to prescribe, and all are surrounded by controversy. Moreover, it is very rare indeed that, with any of our clients, we have any evidence of a physical problem that we are treating with these few physical remedies.

This insecurity has, I believe, led many child and adolescent psychiatrists to push for a greater *medicalisation* of our role. As a result, our understanding of what childhood is – or should be – has become ever narrower, stifling the possibility of difference and colluding with Western culture's intolerance of children. Of course, many cultures struggle with difference, finding it hard to accommodate the alien or outsider. But for the *global* coloniser, imposing a world view – with all its inherent assumptions and definitions, and its intimidating, belittling and pervading sense of inferiority for all who don't fit the powerful coloniser's definition – is something the coloniser need have little awareness of. The colonised either passively accept their inferiority, or bubbles from a seething cauldron of anger and madness emerge.

My intention is not to make a wholesale attack on child and adolescent psychiatry as a discipline, or suggest that as a discipline it should be scrapped. Rather, my aim is to question its assumptions, universals, constructs and resulting clinical practice. As a profession, it is time we appreciated the *relative* nature of the belief systems that we use in our work so that, hopefully, we can make positive use of *other* belief systems. We must reflect on how our position as a dominant and powerful agent in our society can have a profound effect, not only on the clients we work with, but on our modern cultural discourse about children, adolescents and families generally.

POST-MODERN APPROACH

I have found that a post-modern perspective has helped me first to engage in this debate and then to apply it to the work I do. In general terms, a post-modern perspective provides a means for radical questioning of the foundationalism and absolutism of modern conceptions of knowledge. In the field of mental health, this can be interpreted as the idea that no one person or approach has the definitive answer.

Whereas a modernist perspective holds that we are capable of arriving at a universally true, objective reality that separates objective fact from the subjective world, a post-modern perspective turns the focus from exclusively examining apparent exterior objectivity to looking at the subjectivity of the meaning giver.

Modernism privileges a steadily growing body of what it believes to be objective knowledge. And Western modernism – with its ideological belief in fundamental, universal, psychological characteristics common to all humans – is traceable to Western thought as it developed in the early Enlightenment era.

The success of scientific biology – and medical science more generally – has, no doubt, had a big influence on the development of similar universalistic law-discovering approaches to the knowledge base in mental health. However, this approach has been unable to claim the successes seen in other spheres of life; indeed, many believe the very opposite to be true. So, we must finally begin to appreciate that the 'knowledge of the knower' is not a disinterested mental representation of external reality or of some absolute truth.

No longer can we dismiss the potentially different meanings that can be ascribed to similar behaviour and which have a huge impact on the way that we approach our professional practice. We have to appreciate that the belief system we use in child and adolescent psychiatry has developed from goals and values that have been central to Western European civilisation since the Enlightenment. These can no longer be assumed to be universally valid or, indeed, relevant, particularly in the context of the multi-cultural societies in which we now live.

Thus, the post-modern practitioner is no longer the 'expert' who knows how people should behave, think, feel and solve their difficulties. Instead, she or he is committed to a side-by-side, less hierarchical therapeutic relationship in which the practitioner finds ways to honour and privilege the *client's* own abilities and to locate fresh directions and solutions to their problems that incorporate the client's own belief system. The focus is less on what is assumed to be abnormal or pathological, and more on alternatives to a problem-saturated story by careful listening and by responding to the client's own knowledge, with a particular interest being shown in supporting and amplifying clients' strengths and abilities.

In my recent book, *Pathological Child Psychiatry and the Medicalization of Childhood*,[1] I explore how this approach – which involves questioning many fundamental assumptions behind modernist child and adolescent mental health ideologies – can help us, as clinicians, to develop both theoretical and practical ways of grasping the elusive integration nettle. As things stand, too many mental health professions are unnecessarily constrained by an adherence to an increasingly narrow belief system, the agenda of which has been set by drug company assisted biomedical psychiatry. This is potentially problematic with all our clients, but particularly so when dealing with clients from a different cultural background to that of the professional concerned.

WORLD VIEW

Many of the key pathologies in Western developed diagnostic systems have arisen from conceptual constructs influenced by Western philosophical ideas. These so-called pathologies may be absent, nonsensical or have entirely different meanings in cultures where different philosophical traditions have been influential.

Guilt and hopelessness, for example, are cornerstone ideas in the Western construct of depression. Yet symptoms like guilt and hopelessness are unlikely to be relevant for many Buddhists, for whom taking pleasure from things in the world of social relationships is the basis of suffering; consequently, wilful hopelessness and dysphoria can be the first step on the road to salvation. Furthermore, the feeling of 'hope for oneself' is negatively valued in many religious communities and, in any case, is something over which a person may feel they have little autonomy.

Once a professional has been trained, however, and has accepted and identified with a particular professional ideology, then each professional takes that ideology with them and filters the clinical pictures they are faced with through their preferred frameworks. Inevitably, this will challenge the professional's thinking about the cause and treatment of their client's difficulty, into a pre-destined potentially narrow pigeonhole. Yet mainstream conclusions cannot, with our current state of knowledge, represent any ultimate truth because they cannot be confirmed or refuted by verifiable material facts.

FAITH

What is it, then, that keeps professionals believing in the truth of *their* way of understanding the same picture, when there is no way of proving its validity? I think that in the absence of proof, we use faith to sustain our belief in something. We sift through the evidence in a selective way to reinforce our faith and discredit those we feel to be 'non-believers'. In other words, our professional mental health ideologies have been constructed by manipulating evidence to fit the framework, rather than adjusting our frameworks to fit the evidence.

If only we could, as a profession, accept the ideological nature of the belief systems we use. There is nothing shameful about having faith and about needing to believe; it is very human. Faith helps to make sense of the world; for many people, faith falling apart is like their world falling apart. I have come across many clients for whom religion has become much more central following a difficult experience in their lives – for example, refugees fleeing war, torture or other terrifying life events. Faith provides a sense of orientation, continuity and a map with which to structure one's life and make sense of what is happening.

So, what of the system of faith used in modernist child and adolescent psychiatry, with its increasing emphasis on diagnosis and drug treatment? As I attempt to illustrate in my book, when we make a diagnosis we are not discovering the *meaning* of our client's problem; rather, we are giving it our (the professionals') preferred meaning. We are performing a social and political act. And more often than not, we are demonstrating more about our own particular faith, than shedding light on our particular client's problems.

So, we need to ask ourselves, from a political and cultural standpoint, what value systems our particular faith promotes and, therefore, which faith do we wish to promote (and how flexibly)? If we wish to practice in the way that biomedical child and adolescent psychiatry currently does, then we must accept that we are promoting a system whose values are rooted in the Western philosophical Enlightenment – with its emphasis on discovering universal laws, material reality, controlling nature through technical expertise, and a focus on the individual.

We must be prepared to accept its cultural origins in Western history, where medicine has been an active participant in promoting a white, male, middle-class value system which colonised much of the rest of the world, and in the process, suppressed local culture, beliefs, ideologies and practices.

We must also accept that Western biomedical psychiatry represents the economic value system of capitalist, free market thinking and be happy to go along with the pharmaceutical industry's drive to open new markets (children's mental health is a growth area). We must also go along with a short-term perspective on problems and how to solve them, and sign up to the mythical ideal that more production (of knowledge, for example) equates with progress.

And finally, if we wish to sign up to the value system of biomedical psychiatry, we must also understand its political function. Biomedical psychiatry serves governments as one of its agents of social control (a position that sets it apart from the rest of medicine), where so-called treatments to deal with a section of society's 'deviants' are forced on to patients, the vast majority of whom have committed no crime.

CULTURAL VALUES

Eventually, I came to realise that what I had been taught and trained in was a particular faith, a particular system of values, a way of judging people and pathologising them, a way of developing and maintaining a social system – a way of liberating you if you believed in it, a way of terrorising you if you didn't. It was also a way of upholding an economic system, a way of colluding with the elite and the coloniser. Finally, I recognised that I had been trained into belonging to a particular cultural group.

Yet I increasingly found the culture I had been trained into a rather soulless faith with a thin spirituality and, in its fundamentalist form, likely to operate an authoritarian form of social control that marginalises too many experiences. Now, I look back with sadness and pain at how, during my training, I found myself becoming more and more critical of the Arabic culture in which I grew up.

I do not want to see my childhood through any rose tinted spectacles. However, I am still aghast at the arrogance of a psychiatric and psychotherapeutic training that sold me the message that the culture I grew up in was more primitive, less psychologically minded, more cruel and barbarous (particularly to women and children), than the enlightened one I was learning.

Yet in the end, I did not have to go very far to start challenging the assumptions of my training. Which culture is it that is – with good reason – complaining about men who leave their families and their children, bullying, violence, drug abuse, promiscuity, alcohol consumption and suicide (to name but a few) among its young? Which culture is it that is complaining about a lack of collectiveness, poor networks of support and a loss of morals and values? In which culture is it that looking after the self, greed and the accumulation of material commodities has become the main purpose of life? Is this the sign of an advanced, psychologically minded, civilised, compassionate culture?

WHAT OF PSYCHIATRY?

And what of psychiatry, has psychiatry really got anywhere with social suffering? Has it got anywhere with mental pain? On a cultural level, the answer has to be no. In fact, I want to be bold enough to ask if our culture, psychiatry and all, has lost something very valuable about human life with its quest for knowledge, technical expertise and its myth of progress.

In our obsession with compartmentalising human experiences into ever increasing numbers of diagnostic categories, of discovering non-existent genetic anomalies and measuring neurotransmitters in the brain (all of which leads down one blind alley after another), we have lost sight of our common humanity. We have lost sight of a value system that speaks about the common good and that recognises our need for each other, our need to feel connected and our need to belong.

I believe that just as social changes make the biggest difference to the physical health of populations (for example, the huge impact a sewerage system made to public health), it is social changes that can and do make the biggest difference to the mental health of children and adolescents. As a profession, we can contribute to this by engaging in a debate about values, ethics and context.

Challenging the assumptions of current practice can open the door to a genuine effort to integrate diverse perspectives into routine practice and can propel patient, family and local community into the role of expert. As I attempt to illustrate in my book, this does not mean anarchic practising, nor does it mean dispensing with our existing techniques. It does, however, mean developing a new attitude of resistance toward medical hierarchy in a way that allows and celebrates greater creativity, diversity and attention to values and beliefs in our daily clinical practice.

REFERENCE

1 Timimi, S., (2002) *Pathological Child Psychiatry and the Medicalization of Childhood,* Brunner Routledge.

ELEVEN

FOUCAULT AND THE SOCIAL SCIENCES

Madan Sarup

REASON AND UNREASON

[. . .]

In his first well-known book, *Madness and Civilization*,[1] Foucault describes how madness, along with poverty, unemployment and the inability to work, comes in the seventeenth century to be perceived as a 'social problem' which falls within the ambit of responsibility of the state.[1] There is a new conception of the state as preserver and augmenter of the general welfare. In the book there is an important discussion of the emergence of 'humanitarian' attitudes towards the insane at the end of the eighteenth century. The opening of Tuke's Retreat at York and Pinel's liberation of the insane at Bicêtre are portrayed as leading to a 'gigantic moral imprisonment', more oppressive than the former practices of brutal incarceration since they operate on the mind rather than merely on the body.

THE GREAT CONFINEMENT

At the end of the Middle Ages leprosy disappeared from the Western world. Foucault suggests a connection between this and some of the attitudes then taken towards madness. As leprosy vanished a void was created and the moral values had to find another scapegoat. He shows how in the 'classical period' (1500–1800) madness attracted that stigma.

Source: Sarup, M. *An Introductory Guide to Post-Structuralism and Post-Modernism.* Hemel Hempsted: Simon & Schuster, 1993. Reproduced by permission of Pearson Education.

During the Renaissance madmen led an easy, wandering existence. The towns drove them outside their limits and they were allowed to wander in the open countryside. One common way of dealing with the mad was to put them on a ship and entrust them to mariners, because folly, water and sea, as everyone then 'knew', had an affinity with each other. These 'Ships of Fools' were to be found criss-crossing the seas and canals of Europe. Many texts and paintings, for example the works of Breughel, Bosch and Dürer, refer to the theme of madness. These works of art express an enormous anxiety about the relationships between the real and the imaginary. Then, within the space of a hundred years, the 'madship' was replaced by the 'madhouse'; instead of embarkation there was *confinement*. Men did not wait until the seventeenth century to 'shut up' the mad, but it was in this period that they began to 'confine' them.

Why was this? Foucault argues that during the second half of the seventeenth century social sensibility, common to European culture, began to manifest itself; a 'sensibility to poverty and to the duties of assistance, new forms of reaction to the problems of unemployment and idleness, a new ethic of work'.[1] And so, enormous houses of confinement (sometimes called 'houses of correction') were created throughout Europe. To these places a (strangely) mixed group of people, poor vagabonds, the unemployed, the sick, the criminals and the insane were sent. No differentiation was made between them.

Confinement was a massive phenomenon, a 'police' matter whose task was to suppress beggary and idleness as a source of disorder.

The unemployed person was no longer driven away or punished; he was taken in charge, at the expense of the nation but at the cost of his individual liberty. Between him and society an implicit system of obligation was established: he had the right to be fed, but he must accept the physical and moral constraint of confinement.[1]

The repressive function of the houses of confinement was combined with a new use: the internees were made to work. In the Middle Ages the great sin had been pride, in the seventeenth century it was sloth. Since sloth had become the absolute form of rebellion, the idle were forced to work. Labour was instituted as an exercise in moral reform. Confinement played a double role: it absorbed the unemployed in order to mask their poverty and it also avoided the social or political disadvantages of agitation.

In the Renaissance madness had been present everywhere, but the houses of confinement hid it away. Confinement marked a decisive event: 'The new meanings assigned to poverty, the importance given to the obligation to work, and all the ethical values that are linked to labour, ultimately determined the experience of madness and inflected its course.'[1] Most of Foucault's book is a detailed description of how madness was thought about in the seventeenth and eighteenth centuries: he writes about mania and melancholia, hysteria and hypochondria; how it was thought that the savage danger of madness was related to the danger of the passions, and how madness was conceived as a form of animality to be mastered only by discipline.

Gradually in the eighteenth century confinement came to be seen as a gross error; it began to be said that charity was a cause of impoverishment and that vagabonds should seek employment. Moreover, legislators were beginning to be embarrassed because they no longer knew where to place mad people – in prison, hospital or the family. Measured by their functional value alone, the houses of confinement were a failure: when the unemployed were herded into forced-labour shops, there was less work available in neighbouring regions and so unemployment increased. Thus the houses of confinement, a social precaution clumsily formulated by a nascent industrialization, disappeared throughout Europe at the beginning of the nineteenth century.

THE BIRTH OF THE ASYLUM

The legislation passed to segregate criminals and poor people from fools was prompted, as often as not, by a desire to protect the poor and the criminal from the frightening bestiality of the madman. A hallowed tradition has associated Tuke in England and Pinel in France with the liberation of the insane and the abolition of constraint. But, Foucault argues, we must be sceptical of this claim. In fact, Tuke created an asylum where the partial abolition of physical constraint was part of a system whose essential element was the constitution of a self-restraint. 'He substituted for the free terror of madness the stifling anguish of responsibility . . . The asylum no longer punished the madman's guilt, it is true, it did more, it organized that guilt.'[1]

The Quaker Samuel Tuke organized his Retreat so that it had a religious ethos. In it work was imposed as a moral rule, a submission to order. Instead of repression there was surveillance and judgement by 'authority'. Everything at the asylum was arranged so that the insane were transformed into minors and given rewards and punishments like children. A new system of education was applied; first the inmates were to be subjugated, then encouraged, then applied to work: 'The asylum would keep the insane in the imperative fiction of the family; the madman remains a minor, and for a long time reason will retain for him the aspect of the Father.'[1]

During the 'classical period' poverty, laziness, vice and madness mingled in an equal guilt within unreason. Madness during the nineteenth century began to be categorized as social failure. The doctor gained a new social status and increasingly the patient surrendered to the medical profession. In short, the asylum of the age of positivism was not a free realm of observation, diagnosis and therapeutics. In the hands of Tuke and Pinel it became a juridical space where one was accused, judged and condemned – an instrument of moral uniformity. Invoking the names of those who have gone mad, such as Artaud, Hölderlin, Nerval, Nietzsche and Van Gogh, Foucault reminds us that we are in the habit of calling this gigantic moral imprisonment the 'liberation' of the insane.

Foucault's book has a sense of great loss. It states that during the Middle Ages mad people were not locked up; indeed they possessed a certain freedom. There was a notion of the 'wise fool' – like the character in *King Lear*. Even in the eighteenth century madness had still not lost its power; but in the nineteenth century the dialogue between reason and unreason was broken. There is now only the monologue of reason *on* madness. Foucault suggests that there are dimensions that are missing in reason or, to put it in another way, there may be a wisdom in madness.

Human beings have been released from the physical chains, but these have been replaced by mental ones. One of the main themes of the book is how external violence has been replaced by internalization. The birth of the asylum can be seen as an allegory on the constitution of subjectivity. It is an indictment of modern consciousness. *Madness and Civilization* is as much concerned with the plight of everyday consciousness in the modern world as with the specific fate of those labelled insane. Foucault implies that modern forms of public provision and welfare are inseparable from ever tighter forms of social and psychological control. From the beginning, intervention and administrative control have defined the modern state.

According to Foucault madness can never be captured; madness is not exhausted by the concepts we use to describe it. His work contains the Nietzschean idea that there is more to madness than scientific categorization; but in associating freedom with madness he seems to me to romanticize madness. For Foucault, to be free would be *not* to be a rational, conscious being. Though Foucault's position is a relativist one, he actually had deep-seated preferences. Critics of Foucault asked, 'How could Foucault capture the spirit of madness when he was so obviously writing from the viewpoint of reason?'[2] Shouldn't he, logically, have given up writing altogether?

Most of Foucault's books are really analyses of *the process of modernization*. One of the characteristics of his work is the tendency to condense a generally historical argument into a tracing of the emergence of specific institutions. His second main work, *The Birth of the Clinic*, is subtitled 'An Archaeology of Medical Perception'.[3] This perception or 'gaze' is formed by the new, untrammelled type of observation made possible for the doctor at the bedside of the hospitalized patient intersecting with a system of monitoring the state of health of the nation through the new teaching hospital.

Foucault's subsequent books, *The Order of Things* and *The Archaeology of Knowledge*, deal largely with the structure of scientific discourses.[4] (Discourses are perhaps best understood as practices that systematically form the objects of which they speak.) Foucault is concerned with the question, what set of rules permit certain statements to be made?

In *The Order of Things* Foucault argues that in certain empirical forms of knowledge such as biology, psychiatry, medicine, etc., the rhythms of transformation do not follow the continuist schemas of development which are normally accepted. In medicine, for example, within a period of about twenty-five years there arose a completely new way of speaking and seeing. How is it that at certain moments and in certain knowledges there are these sudden transformations? There seem to be changes in the rules of formation of statements which are accepted as scientifically true. There is a whole new 'regime' of discourse which makes possible the separation not of the true from the false but of what may be characterized as scientific from what may not be characterized as scientific.

Unlike most of Foucault's other work, *The Order of Things* and *The Archaeology of Knowledge* are not concerned with the emergence of modern forms of administration. One reason for this may be that the structuralists during the 1960s veered away from any form of political analysis and that he was influenced by them.

Looking back on his early work, Foucault conceded that what was missing was a consideration of the effects of power:

> *When I think back now, I ask myself what else it was that I was talking about, in Madness and Civilization or The Birth of the Clinic, but power? Yet I'm perfectly aware that I scarcely ever used the word and never had such a field of analysis at my disposal.*[5]

In his later work, where Foucault is concerned with power and knowledge, he is much more inclined to talk about 'apparatuses'. An apparatus is a structure of heterogeneous elements such as discourses, laws, institutions, in short, the said as much as the unsaid. The apparatus contains strategies of relations of forces supporting, and supported by, types of knowledge. [. . .]

NOTES

1 M. Foucault, *Madness and Civilization*, London: Tavistock, 1967.
2 Derrida criticized Foucault for still being confined within the structuralist science of investigation through oppositions. See essay entitled 'Cogito and the History of Madness', in J. Derrida, *Writing and Difference*, London: Routledge & Kegan Paul, 1978, p. 34.
3 M. Foucault, *The Birth of the Clinic*, London: Tavistock, 1973.

4 M. Foucault, *The Order of Things*, London: Tavistock, 1970; *The Archaeology of Knowledge*, London: Tavistock, 1972.
5 M. Foucault, *Power/Knowledge: Selected Interviews and Other Writings 1972–1977*, edited by C. Gordon, Brighton: Harvester Press, 1980, p. 115.

PART II

THE WAY THINGS HAPPEN

INTRODUCTION

Janet Seden

The way communications and relationships are experienced in health and social care can, like the weather or the ebb and flow of tides, be unpredictable. The practitioner has to respond to turmoil, changes and crises, encounters that are stormy and those that are calm. The practitioner must understand the particular way the service user responds to events in their life in order to work in a real partnership. Skilled work with events, often referred to as 'process', can create change and make a moment in time positive, and manageable or, if poorly handled, damaging. The way someone communicates and relates influences how each moment is experienced for the other person. This is just as true of relationships which involve little choice for the people involved as it is for those meetings that are chosen.

For health and social care practitioners, attention to the detail of how things happen and the way a relationship develops is at the heart of what they do. Other people's accounts of their experiences offer learning about how to communicate more effectively or insight into what builds positive and empowering relationships. The readings in this part of the book are chosen because in some way they describe or illustrate a situation in someone's life, the meeting with a health or care professional and interactions with other significant people in their lives. The accounts shed light on what service users and workers might identify as skilful or not so skilful ways of communicating and relating.

The poem by Cheryl Palmer, 'Things parents don't say about speech and language therapists', offers a mother's perspective on a meeting where a worker is assessing her child. The use of professional jargon makes it difficult for her to grasp what is meant and Cheryl's unsaid thoughts reflect her concerns. However she stays silent because she needs the service for her child. The poem plays with words and suggests that the communication process is a shifting one with meanings glimpsed and lost. This shows how communication is not a once-and-for-all happening. There are effective and ineffective moments within the same relationship.

When practitioners talk in jargon and use complex or inappropriate words to label others it often goes unchallenged by colleagues, managers and the people who use services. It is perhaps one of the most disempowering forms of 'talk' there is. This theme – the need to check mutual understandings – can be found in many of the accounts in this book. It matters that there is real communicating beyond 'official speak'. Health and social care practitioners need to consider carefully how meaning can be established between two or more people thrown together by the circumstances of needing or providing a care service.

'Eliciting experiences of dementia' by John Killick builds on this theme of learning how to make sense of what other people are saying. 'People with dementia', he says, 'appear to have an urgent need to express feelings that are occasioned by the onset of the condition and that otherwise might remain destructively confined within the psyche.' He shows how by listening to what people with dementia say it is possible to understand the significance of their communications. His way of 'being with' another person gives them assurance that their words still have value (see also 'The experience of dementia' by Tom Kitwood in Part III). Ageing is in itself a process, and Valerie Sinason's poem 'Death of an invisible uncle', gives a personal insight into relating to an older person. A key part of all such communicating and relating is listening and William Isaacs provides more insights into the power of the effective use of this skill in his contribution entitled 'Listening'.

In recent years social policy makers have focused on user views of what makes for a helpful relationship and service. The snippets of website discussion selected under the title of 'What is a good doctor?' illustrate how the quality of what happens between doctor and patient can make a big difference to the patient's perspective on the treatment they received. A good doctor is one who is both medically skilled and human and sensitive. People who use services consistently say that they value respectful attitudes as well as knowledge and skill from health and care professionals.

'One "day" in the life of a hospital out-patient: a patient's perspective' is written by someone who found becoming a patient a scary experience. He reflects on the processes he experienced in hospital and his feelings about the way he was treated. He explains how the hospital systems and procedures for processing patients affected him as much as some of the individual interactions with staff. He also highlights some of the things said and done by professionals that he found 'empowering'. 'Moments in time', edited by Ann Brechin, develops the theme of observing those minute interactions between people which convey respect. Such moments when reflected upon offer a way of appreciating how some ways of communicating and relating are more enhancing than others. They can be studied and used as models. Skilled communication happens in the smallest of interactions between individuals as well as in the larger systemic processes in which individuals are caught up.

Therapy and interviewing, two key activities in care settings, are also based on the process of building relationships through communication. In 'Externalising the problem' Michael White and David Epston describe a therapeutic process with a child and his family. The way the interview is structured helps the people to separate out a particular problem, and the means to address it, from their wider lives and relationships. This allows the family and therapist to focus on 'affirmative action' to problem-solve together. The next three accounts move further into the world of counselling and therapy, where longer appointments and psychotherapeutic processes are examined.

'Counselling for Toads' by Robert de Board is a humorous and accessible representation of what happens in a meeting between therapist and client. The story of Toad going for counselling with Heron is a creative way of illustrating what encountering the 'new world' of therapy can be like. The therapeutic process is explored more seriously in an extract from *The Memory Bird*, a collection of accounts by survivors of sexual abuse, which examines how the therapeutic process can work when it respects, believes and listens to the client's experience or conversely can be disempowering by re-interpreting and labelling. Brenda Nicklinson values flexibility, openness, honesty and genuineness in the therapist as part of the process which takes place for the client. The account by 'Donna' explores this theme further but adds a distinctively black perspective. Donna's narrative describes the risks that exist for a black woman entering therapy, when help is offered by a white therapist, with all the possibilities of abuse of power and misunderstandings.

'Telling other people', edited by Ann Richardson and Dietmar Bolle, slightly shifts the focus. It is still about a process of 'telling', from the service user perspective. However it concentrates on telling your family, friends or others of your HIV and AIDS status. The impact of the different ways this telling happened and the ways the telling was heard and received illuminate different experiences of talking about the same thing, depending on the kinds of relationships and cultural expectations that surround it. These accounts show how much responses matter.

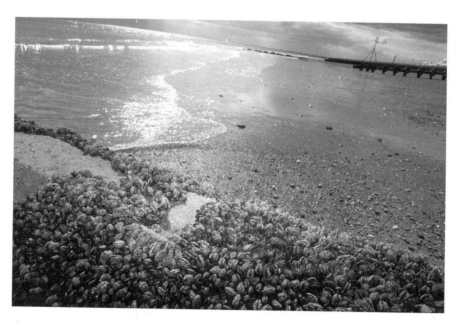

The way communications and relationships are experienced in health and social care can, like the weather or the ebb and flow of tides, be unpredictable. (Image from Third Avenue.)

This part of the book ends with a poem, 'Stat' by Najam Mughal. The work described is part of the structural system of a hospital, in which counting the appointments and the people who keep them reflects the real process which people experience. He claims that 'the fallout of the process between due date and death' is the 'battlefield of main events'. It is a reminder that everyone with a role in health and social care services is part of the event and can make it either caring and positive or negligent and unhelpful. Statistical information gives a 'picture' of what is happening to real people's lives.

When practitioners are involved in communication and relationships developed, abilities to relate carefully and skilfully are a way of giving some power and control back to people, supporting them through relationship, so that each individual experiences respect and dignity rather than an impersonal process. As Mughal says, process is cyclical and never static. Everyone's work contributes to managing human events such as health and illness, births and deaths. As one process ends, 'the process begins again'. Health and social care professionals are constantly communicating and relating alongside what happens in the life events of others.

TWELVE

THINGS PARENTS DON'T SAY ABOUT SPEECH AND LANGUAGE THERAPISTS

Cheryl Palmer

I
It's understandable really –
I mean you can't expect them to go through art school first.

II
So we've been practising every day.

III
It really helped when she explained the controversy about Semantic-Pragmatic Disorder, Asperger's Syndrome and Pragmatic Language Impairment as Dorothy Bishop sees it.

IV
She's only human of course – I suppose she could have had a stressful day herself.

V
You always know where to find her if you need her.

VI
I don't mind whether he enjoys going, so long as she does some accurate tests.

Source: Morley, D (ed.). *The Gift. New writing for the NHS.* Exeter: Stride Publications, 2002.
Reproduced by permission.

VII
Personally I thought she over estimated what my Johnny can do.

VIII
You can really see why they have to do a four year degree course.

IX
And then when he failed on 'not only the bird but also the flower is blue', it suddenly all made sense.

THIRTEEN

ELICITING EXPERIENCES OF DEMENTIA

John Killick

For the past five-and-a-half years, I have been working in nursing homes throughout Britain listening to what people with dementia say. Where permission is granted, I write it down or tape-record the conversation and transcribe it later. All of these texts begin as prose; some end up as poems. At this stage, they exclude my words, which in any case largely take the form of affirmations and various kinds of encouragement. I do some editing. Where there appears to me to be a main theme, I exclude what I judged to be secondary material. It is unnecessary to inject a sense of poetry into these texts: many people with dementia, I have found, display an unforced propensity for metaphor and simile. It is as if the condition had unlocked their imaginative powers while at the same time inhibiting the capacity for logical thought. People with dementia appear to have an urgent need to express feelings that are occasioned by the onset of the condition and that otherwise might remain destructively confined within the psyche. I shall provide a number of examples, with discussion, and conclude with a few observations on procedure.

Here is a woman giving answers to her own questions:

What are we like here?
Well, we're too wide, awake
to be told what to do.

What do I think of it here?
Well, it's better than
working in the wash-house!

Source: Killick, J. *Generations.* Vol. 23, no. 3 (Fall), 1999. Reproduced by permission.

What do people walk like that for?
Well, it's the way
they tighten us off.

How does my eye come out?
Well, it's as flies
going to walk through that door.

Not so long ago such a piece would have been dismissed as nonsense, the proof, if proof were needed, that the speaker was mad. Yet the piece has a tight structure (supplied in this case by the speaker, not by me), and all four verses make a coherent if unconventional whole. In the first, she claims that residents on the trait know what is going on and will not be bossed around. In the second she makes a witty judgement of the establishment, comparing it with a place of traditional hard labour. The third is perhaps the most problematical, but she seems to be articulating cause and effect in relation to the care provided. In the last verse she supplies a vivid metaphor for pain.

In the next poem a man is searching for his wife:

I spend all my time wandering and looking for her.
I'll spend all afternoon up and down
the High Street and up at the Club.

If it was a man you could say 'Sod off!'
Doesn't phone or nothing. You'd think
she was an armored car.

People singing all the time.
Damn nuisance – they're always looking back,
and that's absolute murder.

I haven't eaten and I'm hungry.
I'll go round the corner, crouch
down, and be a grandchild!

He comes across as distressed and somewhat volatile. It is unclear whether his wife is on the unit, or comes to visit him, or is no longer alive. He clearly misses her deeply and is searching for her everywhere. His anger, especially prominent in the second verse, could be the result of frustration. His image of her as an armored car is both funny and alarming. In the third verse he also expresses his intolerance of music, or perhaps it is just the kind of music that is played on the trait. It reminds him of the past, and his concern is with the present. He is also hungry, and in the extraordinary image 'crouch down, and be a grandchild' he dramatically expresses the lengths he would go to obtain a good meal. Or maybe he wants someone to pay attention to him and perceives that people find a child more appealing than an adult.

The next piece is also occasioned by the phenomenon of 'wandering'. The piece is more reflective, but here the speaker identifies the activity as purposeful but cannot detect what purpose it serves. She finds herself being drawn into it almost against her will:

> *Take yourself back to the first time*
> *you saw them doing it.*
> *Hither and thither*
> *and thither and thither*
>
> *It seems definitely*
> *not just absentmindedly.*
>
> *It seems as if*
> *people have something on their mind.*
> *Going from A to B*
> *to C to D to E . . .*
> *They seem to be so restless.*
>
> *I think to myself*
> *they must get awfully tired.*
> *There seems to be*
> *an awful lot of movement.*
>
> *It doesn't strike you at first.*
> *But then everybody's doing it.*
> *It is really rather shattering,*
> *because you've been surprised*
> *by others doing it,*
> *and then you find*
> *that you are doing it yourself!*

The next woman appears to be attempting to articulate either the way she sees the effects of dementia on her mental capacities or the depression from which she may also be suffering:

> *Wear and tear on the mind –*
> *I don't know if I mind it,*
> *that's tricky,*
> *but I know*

wear and tear on the mind –
it suddenly comes on and off
and off and on . . .
Fluctuating . . . dizzymaking . . .

Like the others, this poem is making use of figures of speech. The very idea of the mind suffering attrition is a metaphor – the mind is being considered an item of clothing. The last three lines could be describing a light switch flicked on and off. The poem expresses an emotional state with a remarkable economy of means.

The speaker of the next poem buttonholed me with his urgent requests:

Have you any openings?
Have you got a guide?
Could you come along
And turn a key in a lock for me?

You'll not find my room.
I've only got . . . nothing.

This my room? Not mine.
Not my room.
Not my clothes.
Not my bed.

I'm going home.

Ostensibly, the speaker could be searching for a key to open a door. However, if we take a wider view of the subject of his anxiety, we may see the key as a symbol of coherence and understanding. In this interpretation, perhaps he is looking for the certainties of his life before Alzheimer's struck. The room, the clothes, the bed could be the furniture of his mind, furniture that has not just been rearranged by the condition but removed. The poignant intensity of his appeals may come from the realization that he has no 'home' to go to any more.

Here is a woman who appears to be expressing a comparable state of mind:

I have a problem:
I have a house on either side of the road,
but I only have a room in one of them.
How do I cross the busy road?
And what happens if I break down in the middle?

I have another problem:
I've spilt something on my skirt.
There's nothing there?
Are you sure there's nothing there?
Well it must have been in another room.
Well is must have been in the other house.
Well it must have been another skirt.

And I have a problem about kindness:
A lot of those who come round here
are not interested in being kind to others.
Kind is the only thing one can do here.
It is all there is that can help.
I don't try to be it.
You shouldn't have to try to be kind.

The first verse partakes of the rawness of existential distress. Maybe the two houses symbolize the before and after dementia in relation to the woman's mental faculties. Maybe they are real houses, the home she used to live in and the institution where she is now. But she also uses the term 'break down' of the process of traveling from one to the other, which can have more than one interpretation. The second verse deals with a problem of a more trivial nature. Or is it? Why should she go to such extravagant lengths to assert that the stain is indeed there? Could it be that she feels in some way besmirched by circumstances? The third verse breaks through to the clarity of a major statement: this is what people in her condition need, she is saying. She precisely defines what is required and how so many people fall short of this standard. It is both chastening and energizing to be receiving this message out of the mouth of a person with dementia.

My final example comes from a woman who at first appeared withdrawn but then warmed to the idea of talking out of her inner self. This is an excerpted version of her poem:

You give it as you talk.
There's no-one saying it
or doing it in a certain time.
You take it and make it your own.

There have been other loves but none
like that of my mother.
She had birds that came onto her hand,
pecked,
and flew away.

What a wonderful time! –
we were brought up that way.

She was very particular
how and where. I shall not forget.
She would make little noises
and then pull it in –
the string of humankindness . . .

Twice and twice over
what I think is important.
My hiding place now is one
that I can stretch out to
and run away to for a while.

The first verse is rather mysterious. It seems to be concerned with gaining access to a private world. The speaker may be saying that you have to do this in your own time and at your own pace. Then comes the description of her mother. It is full of tenderness and ends with a remarkable metaphor – the way her mother drew other people toward her into the circle of her love, like winding in a ball of string. The final extract seems to be an important statement about owning one's own experience. First of all she asserts her right to it, and then she reveals how she is able to reach it on occasion. This part reveals the power of memory and how it is something to cherish and not necessarily to share, even though she has been extraordinarily generous in permitting me a glimpse of her treasures on this occasion.

At this point, I can anticipate a question from my readers: What must you do to achieve such a level of rapport with a person? My answer is that you do not have to do anything special or be anyone special. You do, however, have to develop the qualities of empathy and self-effacement and to learn to keep silent. It is so easy to fill the gaps between speech with idle chatter. This temptation must be resisted so that the person with dementia has time and space to decide what to say and how to articulate it. So must the propensity to ask questions. You are not conducting an interview but engaging in a dialogue – a dialogue in which your companion must have the lion's share of the lines.

And you cannot rush into a relationship and expect intimacies to unfold (that is true of any relationship, after all). You have to patiently build the interaction until the other person feels relaxed and trust has been established. With some people, that can take a few minutes, with some a few hours, with others a number of visits. And you have to give of yourself continually, using eye contact, body language, and touch as well as speech.

Remember, you are not setting an agenda, you are being with the person. It therefore follows that you are not engaged in a reminiscence activity. If the person does not wish to speak of the past, he or she will not do so. It is unhelpful also, to know much about the person's past, which only provides the temptation to raise particular issues. Of course, if you have had a number of conversations with a person, you may have gleaned some information about the person's life, but that is only what the person had chosen to vouchsafe to you, not what you have gleaned from others or a care plan. Prior knowledge creates power in a relationship, and it is important in these special circumstances not to add to the imbalances that already inevitably exist. So far as possible, you should attempt to ensure that in this particular, you and the person with dementia proceed on an equal footing.

You must seek the individual's permission before you share any insights gained with others, whether in the individual's immediate circle or in the world beyond. Having their words written down is empowering for people with dementia. It affirms their dignity and gives an assurance that their words still have value. Some individuals positively desire a sharing process: One woman said, 'Anything you can tell people about how things are for me is important.'

It is the same woman who also remarked 'It's a mm do, this growing ancient ... The brilliance of my brain has slipped away when I wasn't looking.'

All poems are by residents of Westminster Health Care nursing homes, where the author has been writing in residence for the past six years.

FOURTEEN

DEATH OF AN INVISIBLE UNCLE

Valerie Sinason

Uncle smiles faintly and lives in an armchair
and if he holds up the Daily Mirror
he is invisible

We are playing cowboys and Indians,
whooping and war dancing around
the totem pole of his silence

and Uncle in the Armchair lives, we think,
because of the smoke signals rising
behind newspaper rock,
the semaphore of his blind pipe tapping
and the slow movement of the gold tobacco tin.

Uncle in the armchair
my invisible uncle,
my four word 'hello', 'goodbye,' 'you've grown' uncle
who slipped sticky sixpences to the nieces and nephews
who never knew his views
save that buttons were not sewn on suits
properly nowadays.

Uncle sewed and sewed in the sweatshops
rows of buttons in stitches of beauty

Source: Sinason, V. Inkstains & Stilletos. West Kirby, Wirral: Headland, 1987.
Reproduced by permission.

that nobody could see
and gentlemen's jackets and suits of velvet
for the scratched dummy in the hot back room.

Now he faces me always
his bald head downwards
not a stitch in sight
not a hook of hair
and his newspaper face turned inwards
and his anger a slow stitch rising.

And on the day the invisible man became visible
on the day his anger burst through
the exquisite stitching of veins
on the day his soul cried out for a velvet suit

On the day he exploded in a red volcano of buttons
on the day his armchair gaped like an empty hanger

he died
and became invisible again

And the relatives cried for the living only
leaving his name
to the tailor of stone
and the cold embroidery of earth.

FIFTEEN

LISTENING

William Isaacs

The heart of dialogue is a simple but profound capacity to listen. Listening requires we not only hear the words, but also embrace, accept, and gradually let go of our own inner clamouring. As we explore it, we discover that listening is an expansive activity. It gives us a way to perceive more directly the ways we participate in the world around us.

This means listening not only to others but also to ourselves and our own reactions. Recently a manager in a program I was leading told me, 'You know, I have always prepared myself to speak. But I have never prepared myself to listen.' This is, I have found, a common condition. For listening, a subject we often take for granted, is actually very hard to do, and we are rarely prepared for it. Krishnamurti, the Indian philosopher, put the challenge this way:

> I do not know if you have ever examined how you listen, it doesn't matter to what, whether to a bird, to the wind in the leaves, to the rushing waters, or how you listen in a dialogue with yourself, to your conversation in various relationships with your intimate friends, your wife or husband. If we try to listen we find it extraordinarily difficult, because we are always projecting our opinions and ideas, our prejudices, our background, our inclinations, our impulses; when they dominate, we hardly listen at all to what is being said. In that state there is no value at all. One listens and therefore learns, only in a state of attention, a state of silence, in which this whole background is in abeyance, is quiet; then, it seems to me, it is possible to communicate.

Source: Isaacs, W. *Dialogue and the Art of Thinking Together*. New York: Random House inc., 1999. Reproduced by permission.

To listen is to develop an inner silence. This is not a familiar habit for most of us. Emerson once joked that ninety-five per cent of what goes on in our minds is none of our business! We often pay great attention to what goes on in us, when what is actually required is a kind of disciplined self-forgetting. This does not have to be difficult. It is within the reach of each of us.

To do this you do not have to retreat to a monastery or to be converted to some new belief. You do, though, have to do some deliberate work to cultivate settings inside yourself and with others – where it is possible to listen. In other words, you must create a space in which listening can occur.

The ways we have learned to listen, to impose or apply meaning to the world, are very much a function of our mental models, of what we hold in our minds as truths. But the physical functioning of our ears, and how they differ from other senses, can shed light on how we can learn to 'make sense' in new ways.

THE SENSE OF HEARING

The sense of hearing is ever present. You cannot turn it off; there is no switch. You can close your eyes. You can become less sensitive to or even limit your sense of touch, or taste, or smell. But unless you are deaf (or becoming deaf), you cannot stop yourself from hearing without external aid.

In her book *A Natural History of the Senses*, Diane Ackerman says that hearing's job is:

> *Partly spatial. A gently swishing field of grain that seems to surround one in an earthly whisper doesn't have the urgency of a panther growling behind and to the right. Sounds have to be located in space, identified by type, intensity, and other features. There is a geographical quality to listening.*

Our hearing puts us on the map. It balances us. Our sense of balance is intimately tied to our hearing; both come from the same source within our bodies. We listen in a way that tells us about the dimensionality of our world. Hearing is *auditory*, of course, relating to sound. The words 'auditory' and 'oral' have the same roots as the word *audience* and *auditorium*. Their most ancient root means 'to place perceptions'. When we listen, we place our perceptions.

Our culture, though, is dominated by sight. We see thousands of images flashed across our minds in an hour of television or the Internet. The result of this external bombardment of visual impressions is that we tend now to think in these ways. In the Western world we have begun to be habituated to this quick pace, and are impatient with other rhythms. But seeing and listening are very different.

The substance of seeing is light. Light moves at a far more rapid pace than sound: 186,000 miles per second as opposed to 1,100 feet per second. To listen, in other words, you must *slow down* and operate at the speed of sound rather than at the speed of light.

The eye seems to perceive at a superficial level, at the level of reflected light. While the eye sees at the surface, the ear tends to penetrate below the surface. In his book *Nada Brohmn: The World Is Sound: Music and the Landscape of Consciousness*, Joachim-Ernst Berendt points out that the ear is the only sense that fuses an ability to measure with an ability to judge. We can discern different colours, but we can give a precise *number* to different sounds. Our eyes do not let us perceive with this kind of precision. An unmusical person can recognise an octave and, perhaps once instructed, a quality of tone, that is a C or an F-sharp. Berendt points out that there are few 'acoustical illusions' – something sounding like something that in fact it is not – while there are many optical illusions. The ears do not lie. The sense of hearing gives us a remarkable connection with the invisible, underlying order of things. Through our ears we gain access to vibration, which underlies everything around us. The sense of tone and music in another's voice gives us an enormous amount of information about that person, about their stance toward life, about their intentions.

To listen well, we must attend both to the words and the silence between the words. I once held a dialogue retreat in Amsterdam with a group of consultants, managers, and civic leaders. On the first day, people were quite frustrated and contentious: some found the conversation going too slowly, others felt there seemed to be no coherent theme. People developed many different opinions about what was happening and what ought to happen. The afternoon of the second day I opened the proceedings by simply asking people to reflect on the day's events. To people's surprise, there was a profound silence. The silence filled the room like a rest between the notes. The silence seemed to take us in, bring us alive, evoking a profound state of listening. In that state all one's words feel inadequate, almost an imposition. Slowly people began to put their thoughts into words. Many later reported that like a jazz ensemble playing together, they felt they had to improvise, that all of their previous ideas seemed out of place. They tried to speak in a way that matched the intensity of the silence.

LISTENING AND THE PRINCIPLE OF PARTICIPATION

Our capacity to listen puts us in contact with the wider dimensions of the world in which we live. It lets us connect to it. Listening can open in us a door, a greater sense of participation in the world. I see listening, properly understood and developed, as an immediate gateway that can connect us with the much-touted but much-misunderstood notion that we live in a 'participative universe', one of the four key principles that underlie the approach to dialogue proposed in this book.

The principle of participation builds upon the realization that individuals are active participants in the living world, a part of nature as well as observers of it. At the heart of the matter here is the idea that human beings participate intimately in their worlds and are not separate from them.

Ideas like these fly directly in the face of what science has told us about the world over the last three hundred years. We have had the belief that man was separate from nature and needed to control it. Descartes, in many ways the founder of modern rationalism, declared in the seventeenth century that there was an absolute split between thinking man and the world he observes. Today, what we call 'real' are the things we can quantify and measure objectively – views stemming directly from Descartes and the canon of modern science that grew from it – 'specific location'. This idea is simply that if you cannot find a precise measurement and location for something, it does not really exist.

There is clearly validity to this perspective at the physical level of things. But it gets more problematic as we move into thoughts and feelings. Science now has attempted to help us 'locate' our thoughts by conducting brain scans; but as I indicated earlier, this tells us only about the external surface, not the interior contours of our thought.

The principle of participation that lies behind the practice of listening is well demonstrated by a hologram. A hologram is a three-dimensional image created by the interference pattern of two interacting laser beams. This interference pattern is captured on photographic film or a holographic plate. When a laser is directed at this special plate, it produces a three-dimensional reproduction of the image that was recorded.

All the information contained on the plate is enfolded into every part of the plate. For instance, if you were to break this plate up into smaller pieces and shine the laser through it, you would still see the whole image. As the pieces of the plate get smaller, the image becomes dimmer and more diffuse as well; there is less information on it. The density of information on the original plate made the image bright and clear. But every piece of the holographic plate contains the whole image. Similarly, as David Bohm argued, information about the whole of the universe is 'enfolded', or contained, in each part.

To get a sense of how this might work, consider the experience of listening to music. Music acts in a slightly different way. Music, too, is experienced as a living whole. Though any one note may be discerned individually, it is held in the context of reverberations of the notes that came before and the anticipation of those that will follow. Each part of the music contains information about the whole piece. If we heard one note at a time, we would not tend to think of this as music. Bohm suggests that the universe itself is like this: each part is enfolded into every other part. There is a surface-level order that has only a relative independence, like the individual notes of a piece of music. Everything is interconnected.

We are part of a much larger universe in ways that may continue to surprise us. Henri Bortoft tells us in his book *The Wholeness of Nature* that the night sky is also enfolded in each aspect of it:

> *We see this night time world by means of the light 'carrying' the stars to us, which means that this vast expanse of sky must all be present in the light which passes through the small hole of the pupil into the eye. Furthermore, other observers in different locations can see the same expanse of night sky. Hence we can say that the stars seen in the heavens are all present in the light which is at any eye-point. The totality is contained in each small region of space, and when we use optical instruments like a telescope, we simply reclaim more of that light.*

A telescope focuses the light, making the holographic image brighter and stronger.

LANGUAGE IS HOLOGRAPHIC

Our language is also holographic. Each word contains not only the wider context of paragraph and sentence but the deeper context of our lives. When you first interact with someone, their initial words carry the entire hologram of their consciousness to you. The full meaning might not be completely clear to you initially since the information may not be focused enough – like seeing without a telescope, not enough light has been captured to let you see what is actually there. But when you know someone for a long time, or have a close relationship, the richness of the information changes. I can remember hearing my mother say my name at different times while I was growing up and knowing that just that one word could mean anything from 'I want you to do something for me' to 'You are in big trouble.' Most of the time I knew precisely which it was. These meanings, and many others, were enfolded in me and her and influenced how we both interacted.

Every part of ourselves is enfolded in every part of our conversations whether we realize it or not. But we cannot always tell the extent of our participation. There is not enough information to produce a clear and coherent understanding. We lack a focusing process – a way of containing the enormity in a small space. Dialogue is the focusing mechanism for the hologram of conversation. Through it we can expand our awareness to include ever-greater wholeness. Dialogue is a process that can allow us to become aware of our participation in a much wider whole. Like the telescope, it focuses the available light more completely so that we can see more.

THE EARTH LISTENS TO US

The mechanistic view of life that we have inherited tells us that the world is an objectively existing, separate place. We hear the sounds of the world. But this view of things is quite insular. In preparing ourselves for dialogue, it is helpful to recall that there was a time when human beings were much more intimately involved in the landscape, where our very language mimicked and was developed from the music of the earth itself. We not only listen to the earth; it listens to us.

Writer David Abram, in his book *The Spell of the Sensuous*, outlines the ways in which human language was deeply rooted in the physical sounds of the earth – the birds, the forces of weather, the rivers. To the indigenous peoples, the earth itself spoke. Oral cultures had a deep attunement with the nuances of their physical surroundings. It was the arrival of written language, according to Abram, that gradually marked a shift away from human beings feeling that they are participants with the earth, toward a more objective stance.

When someone claims that his indigenous ancestors had a more intimate connection with the earth than he does, this may seem quaint to modern, sophisticated ears. The idea that the earth 'spoke' to the indigenous peoples may fit into one's picture of an earlier animistic culture – one in which all of nature was endowed with conscious life. But most would not see it as anything more than that – a belief – that science has long since disproved.

But notice: when you read these words, it is very likely that you are hearing them inside your head as you go along. The words of our written language *speak to us*. We endow them with voices. They come alive. We enter into a strange, almost dreamlike state with the words. Says Abram,

Our senses are now coupled, synaesthetically, to these printed shapes as profoundly as they were once wedded to cedar trees, ravens, and the moon. As the hills and the bending grasses once spoke to our tribal ancestors, so these written letters and words now speak to us.

Animism is not dead; it has just changed form. It is in fact a fundamental human capacity – our ability to let our senses fuse with the world around us and so enable us to participate directly in it.

Through a detailed process that Abram traces in his book, this capacity has gradually been redirected toward written language.

LEARNING TO LISTEN

Learning to listen begins with recognizing how you are listening now. Generally, we are not all that conscious of how we listen. You can begin to listen by listening first to yourself and to your own reactions. Ask yourself, What do I feel here? Or How does this feel? Try to identify what you feel more carefully and directly. Beginning with the perception of your own feelings connects you to your heart and to the heart of your experience. To learn to be present, we must learn to notice what we are feeling now.

BE AWARE OF THOUGHT

As you begin to listen, you can also begin to notice what you are thinking. Focus your thoughts on someone you care about for a moment. Almost immediately, you may find that you are flooded with thoughts and images of that person. You may also experience a range of feelings. Your memory plays a very powerful force in how you perceive those around you.

To listen is to realize that much of our reaction to others comes from memory; it is stored reaction, not fresh response at all. Listening from my predispositions in this way is *listening from the 'net' of thought* that I cast on a particular situation.

Let me give you an analogy. England has been inhabited continuously for many centuries. A large number of people occupy a relatively small geographic space. As a result, almost every corner, every piece of land, is settled, cultivated, occupied. There is a certain density to people's memories about this place, and you can feel this as you travel in the country. It is not a land of wide-open spaces that have yet to be explored fully. Here you get the sense that everything has been explored very fully for a very long time. It is rich as a result. Every stone in every building has many stories it could tell compared to, say, a stone in rural Nevada.

The landscape of our listening works in similar ways. We know well and have explored fully certain parts of our inner lives. Listening in this mode, from the net of our thought, from this rich background, may make us feel quite clever. After all, we seem to know a lot about what is being said, have things to say, reactions to express, opinions to voice. But just as a densely populated area like England can feel claustrophobic, this kind of listening is not always very expansive. This net of our thought, however finely woven, is still based on memory. It is limited, even unintelligent, in the sense that it cannot respond in a new way to what is happening. The word *intelligence* is quite revealing on this score. It comes from two Latin roots, *inter* and *legere*, which mean 'to gather between'. Intelligence, then, is the active, fresh capacity to think, to gather between already existing categories. In other words, we can learn to listen either from the net we already have, or to the spaces between.

'Be aware of thought' was a piece of advice Krishnamurti often offered. He would ask someone, 'Why do you walk that way?' And they might respond, 'Because I do.' He would retort, 'Well, that's your thought.' To be aware of thought is to learn to watch how our thoughts dictate to us much of our personal and collective experience. Much of what human beings do happens simply by virtue of our agreements that it should. By agreement alone – not because there is any particular reason, some countries drive on the left and others on the right, for instance. What do you do that is simply your thought?

STICK TO THE FACTS

A common joke about someone who has an overinflated sense of himself is 'He is a legend in his own mind.' We need to learn to listen with a great deal more humility. This typically means literally coming down to earth and connecting what we think with the experiences that lead us to think it. While this may seem obvious and easy, in practice people continually jump to conclusions, speak abstractly, and fail to notice they are doing so. A new discipline of listening to what is said can make a real change.

This is not always so easy to do. We are often unaware of the extent to which we assume what we see is what is there. A colleague of mine tells the story of a man who went one day to pick up his high-school-age daughter and another girl. As he drove up to the place he was to meet her, he saw her leaning on a black BMW sedan. Standing nearby were two young men, both with pagers and cell phones. One had a ponytail. This man's immediate thought: drug dealers! But he noticed how he had begun to judge them, and stopped himself. He went up and started to talk to them, and found that they were volunteer firemen, that the BMW was used and much older than he had realized, and that the young men were very gentle, very bright, and capable.

As they were driving away, his daughter's friend burst into tears. When asked what was wrong, she said, 'I wish my parents would talk to me the way you just talked to them.'

THE LADDER OF INFERENCE

We need to distinguish between the inferences we make about experience and the experience itself. One powerful tool for helping to do this is called the Ladder of Inference. This tool, developed by Chris Argyris, a professor at Harvard, is a simple model of how we think. It suggests that what we experience we process and create inferences about our experience, typically at lightning speed, without noticing that we are doing so. What we do not notice principally is the difference between a direct experience and our assessment of it.

For instance, if I called a meeting for two and someone showed up at two-thirty, several people might think to themselves, 'She's late.' Someone else might further think that she did not care about the meeting. A third person might say, 'She is always late on Thursdays.' All of this happens in milliseconds: the assessments are made, the reactions are in, it all seems obvious and true. But is it? In what ways?

We draw conclusions like these all the time. Our conclusions have the simple reasoning that 'this is the way it is'. But I have found that these sorts of conclusions are never fully accurate.

For instance, in the story above, what is the directly observable data? Many people would say it is the fact that she was late. But is late really directly observable data?

Can you see, touch, smell, hear, or feel 'late'? 'Well, yes,' a student once replied to this question. 'The clock says two-thirty, the meeting started at two, she's late! What's the discussion about?' he exploded. Gradually, we explored the idea that 'late' is an inference drawn from the fact of the clock striking two-thirty, a foot crossing the threshold, a prior statement about the meeting time, and an agreement to meet. People sometimes hear this as doubting whether this person is late. I am sure she was, *by the standards of our community*. But that is a long way from saying that is an observable fact. It may be a valid judgment.

Why is this important? One of the ways we sustain the culture of thinking alone is that we form conclusions and then do not test them, treating our initial inferences as facts. We wall ourselves off, in other words, from the roots of our own thinking. And when we are invested in an opinion, we tend to seek evidence that we are right and avoid evidence that we are wrong.

REFERENCES

David Abram, *The Spell of the Sensuous*, New York: Pantheon, 1996, p. 138.

Diane Ackerman (1990) *A Natural History of the Senses*, New York: Vintage Books, p. 178.

David Bohm and Basil Hiley (1993) *The Undivided Universe*, London: Routledge, p. 382.

Henri Borftoft, *The Wholeness of Nature*, Hudson, NY: Lindisfarne Press, 1996, p. 5.

Jiddu Krishnamurti (1968) *Talks and Dialogues*, New York: Avon Books.

SIXTEEN

WHAT IS A GOOD DOCTOR?

Letters from the BMJ website

THE DOCTOR'S DOCTOR 28 JUNE 2002

A. H. Tay, Paediatrician, Alpha Baby and Child Specialist
A 'good' doctor is one to whom I'd entrust my own health, or that of my loved ones. The qualities I'd like to see in such a doctor include a genuine concern for patients, good communication skills, a willingness to listen, and open-mindedness, with a readiness to admit uncertainties and/or the need for help from others.

I don't think it is possible to 'make' medical students or young doctors care for their patients, but I think they can certainly be encouraged and inspired by examples from their teachers and mentors.

Communication skills need to be emphasised early in the training process. I have observed that even among doctors who are caring and competent there is frequently a failure of communication with the patient, at a level that the average layman can understand.

WHO IS A GOOD DOCTOR? 28 JUNE 2002

Om Prakash, Head, Medicine Department, St Martha's Hospital, Bangalore, India
A good doctor is one who combines heart and head.

He almost always places wisdom before intelligence and looks at the patient with kind eyes filled with empathy. He intuitively knows that he likes people, with all their idiosyncrasies and tantrums and treats them like children.

A good doctor updates his knowledge often and keeps a track of notable update programs. He also takes care that he can separate the wheat from the chaff in many journal articles!

AFTER HIPPOCRATES 28 JUNE 2002

Rita Pal, Writer and Campaigner
The art of medicine has come into disrepute simply because our medical schools fail to select the doctors who will make the best clinicians, a regulation body that is constantly seen to allow doctors to deviate from the Hippocratic Oath and an establishment who is now out of touch with the true art of medicine.

One can mix all this into a broth of journalists who have no concept of medicine and spout what they wish and you have the ingredients of hysteria.

The essence of a good doctor is one who is selfless, one whose patient becomes the priority in order to uphold the art of medicine. Medical students who are good communicators are not necessarily high-flying academics. Academia is often confused with doctors who understand patients. The problem-solving approach is vital as a doctor is faced with unpredictable situations. The medical culture has to open its doors to sixth formers from all walks of life, who are able to show empathy, who are able to talk at the level of the patient and who are able to make management decisions after respecting the person's autonomy. Often communication problems lead to disastrous consequences. There are many doctors who have no empathy with those from different walks of life, e.g. prostitutes, those with a disability, the elderly and people from ethnic environments. Education in humanity is a crucial part in creating a good doctor.

Adherence to the Hippocratic Oath is the main ingredient of a good doctor. A good doctor is one who is prepared to sacrifice all for the welfare of his or her patient. This is rare and almost extinct in a modern world where many other commodities seem to take priority.

HOW TO MAKE A REALLY GOOD DOCTOR 29 JUNE 2002

Robert I. Rudolph, MD, FACP, Clinical Professor of Dermatology, University of Pennsylvania School of Medicine, USA
Aside from the obvious ones of a fine medical school, great teachers, and lots of hands on clinical experience, I think the very best way to produce a

good (read sympathetic and humane) doctor is to force the student-doctor or Resident to become a patient. I feel every doctor in pupa should have many tubes of blood drawn over a few days by poor phlebotomists, have an NG tube inserted once or twice, undergo a thorough sigmoidoscopy, barium enema and bowel prep, and perhaps even be made to spend a night or two confined to a hospital bed, plugged into an IV, and then be subjected to harried and uncaring staff physicians and/or nurses while bed-ridden.

I'll bet a case of wine that this trenchant exercise will produce far more empathetic, sympathetic, and good doctors than multiple lectures on sensitivity and humanism by some medical academic, ethics professor, or member of the cloth.

I daresay that I truly believe that my 'being a patient' experiences as a student sure as hell helped mould me into the caring and sensitive practitioner I am today!

A GOOD DOCTOR IS COMPETENT AND COURTEOUS 2 JULY 2002

Jean A. Leyland, Research Nurse, Department of Oncology, University of Cambridge/Addenbrooke's Hospital, Cambridge
In my experience both as a colleague (nurse, midwife, health visitor, researcher, nurse manager and Regional Nurse), and as a patient, I think a good doctor:

> Is a team player who gets to know the team, their skills and experience, remembers their names, etc.
>
> Works with their colleagues, e.g. the doctor who calls in a colleague when he is puzzled, the GP who works in partnership with the Health Visitor to tackle post-natal depression, the A&E consultant who holds regular team de-briefings, the doctor who recognises a colleague's special skills and interests and nurtures them.
>
> Is a good teacher, leader, coach, mentor and student all his/her life.
>
> Is courteous and thoughtful (being told to strip to the waist and wait for the breast surgeon to appear is just plain rude).
>
> Looks as though they are pleased to see you.
>
> Listens, shows interest and relates to you as an individual.
>
> Has read your notes before a follow-up consultation begins.
>
> Asks your opinion and respects your views and feelings.
>
> Does not treat you as a fool (my mother had a colectomy for cancer, an operation that her surgeon described as 'taking a little bit out of your bottom').

Demonstrates competence and keeps up to date (being prescribed a drug referred to in last week's medical press as 'quite inappropriate' is frightening).
Involves you in the decision-making process.
Is kind, gentle and sympathetic when you are feeling awful, especially when you are in pain.

Contrary to what some of the doctors I have met in my 30-plus years in nursing believe, a good doctor is not necessarily one who:

Is rude and arrogant to colleagues and patients alike.
Is always late for NHS commitments.
Makes mistakes but doesn't say sorry.
Has the longest list of publications.
Has the most beds.
Dresses as though he or she has never touched a patient in their lives.
Thinks they know it all.

In short, a good doctor is competent and courteous, and enjoys being a doctor. Just as we all should be in our chosen work. Not much to ask, is it?

SEVENTEEN

ONE 'DAY' IN THE LIFE OF A HOSPITAL OUT-PATIENT: A PATIENT'S PERSPECTIVE

Anonymous

Bill developed cancer, which was successfully treated. The following vignettes illustrate some typical and 'normal' communication and inter-action issues in the context of excellent polices and practices in health care. (When practices are good the issues are clearer.)

1 REFERRAL NETWORKS/HELP-SEEKING BEHAVIOUR

Bill became aware that he had a health problem but delayed seeking medical advice for nearly a year. The reasons for the delay included several obstacles:

> two of his friends were dying of cancer at this time
> he had to negotiate disability access
> he had some responsibilities for an elderly relative
> he was frightened
> he wanted to finish some professional work.

He eventually booked an appointment with his GP, and could have walked away a hundred times from the surgery. He obviously felt very guilty and scared.

Issue: social and psychological factors are as significant as physical ones in health care (whole person issue). Bill was afraid that the doctors would shout at him for his prevarication, but his fears were groundless. One of his friends, though, had been harshly critical of his behaviour, saying that it was his duty and obligation to seek early medical help. Bill said that he would have if he could have! Bill was seen by a consultant within one week and treatment and tests started immediately.

2 THE FIRST CONSULTATION

Bill was obviously apprehensive – even frightened – but he wanted to behave well and to be a 'good patient'.

The consultant asked some routine questions.

He then asked Bill if he was employed.

Bill was furious because he was proud (but not vainglorious) of his professional career, and hadn't he detailed this on his admission sheet!

Issue: the consultant probably used this question as a means of engaging with the patient, whereas Bill interpreted the question 'too rationally'. The communication backfired although the parties got on track once more.

3 THE SECOND CONSULTATION

The consultant shook Bill's hand and acknowledged one of their (mutual) colleagues.

A medical student had taken Bill's history:

he took this standing up
he was slightly judgemental, i.e. expressing dismay and surprise about Bill's delay in seeking medical help. Bill felt guilty; after all he had not behaved according to his own model of help-seeking behaviour.

Issues: the patient was feeling frightened and vulnerable but wanted to be helpful although he knew he would have to divulge many personal details.

The student was probably as anxious and nervous as Bill.

Bill invited the student to take a seat (thereby stepping out of role) but he would not.

4 THE AMBULANCE SERVICE

Arrangements were eventually made for Bill to undergo a five-week course of radiotherapy. There were discussions about how he would reach the clinic, and the consultant eventually suggested hospital transport. Bill was pleased about this because he wanted to be as independent as possible in the circumstances; his family and friends had been extremely supportive.

Bill observed some patients becoming very upset because they had had to wait for the ambulance; they were not treated immediately on arrival at the clinic; and they had to wait again to be transported home.

Issues: the ambulance service is neither a taxi service nor a chauffeur service; it is a hospital transport system. Patients are members of three cohorts:

1   to be transported to the clinic
2   to be treated
3   to be transported home.

Bill's transport took about four hours, sometimes less, sometimes more. Once he worked out the system, he felt less anxious and distressed. (Knowing may not always reduce stress.)

5 'LOST' IN THE CLINIC

Fairly early on in his radiotherapy treatment, Bill was 'lost' in the clinic. He had been waiting four hours and the only person who noticed he was still there was a volunteer worker. Eventually, one of the radiotherapists wondered why Bill was still at the clinic. Bill explained that he was determined not to complain or make a fuss – he was proud to be an NHS patient. The therapist said Bill should have complained and must do so if necessary in future.

Issue: the issue was a systemic one rather than the fault of any individual.

There was a temporary receptionist on duty who failed to complete a normal routine.

There was a change of shifts, so another routine was missed.

Bill was caught between these systems.

The clinic staff were mortified. Bill had an interesting discussion with them about systems approaches in health care! (In an American psychiatric hospital cycles of incontinence in patients were traceable to patterns of communication between staff; Stanton and Schwartz, 1954.)

6 DEFENCE STRATEGIES/MECHANISMS

From any perspective (behavioural, cognitive, psychodynamic, humanist, etc.) being diagnosed with cancer is traumatic. By definition Bill was unaware of his unconscious reactions. Although his cancer was not terminal, death is always 'on the cards' in these circumstances. Bill was not morbid or overwhelmed by thoughts of his own mortality, although such preoccupations were ever around him. Occasionally, thoughts or feelings about the 'enormity' of it all invaded him, but soon passed. Two of his friends had recently died of cancer. Bill's GP had helpfully observed that every case was different. Bill was reassured by this, as he was by the GP's statement that 'all was not lost'.

When Bill went to the clinic for the results of various tests he felt he was climbing a scaffold; he was dreading seeing the consultant.

He was elated to be told that all the test results were clear (i.e. no secondaries) although he still had cancer.

The following day Bill was besieged by a (classic) panic attack, thinking that the consultant might have withheld information or not told him the truth. This feeling of panic soon passed and equilibrium was restored.

There are no inevitable stages of coping with these situations, although Bill was able to resume a valued lifestyle. He sometimes switched from being anxious and fed up to being detached but these feelings were short-lived.

Tasks and coping

Tasks

Learn the requirements for restoring bodily functions.
Maintain self-esteem.
Handle recurring negative emotions.
Maintain a valued lifestyle.
Keep in touch with family and friends.
(Coelho *et al.*, 1974; Moos and Tsu, 1977)

Coping

Coping strategies: physical, psychological and social.
Coping styles: learn how to cope with threats to life, etc.; adopt different kinds of illness roles.

7 COMMUNICATION/EMPOWERMENT

A health care worker asks a new mother to name the worst thing she can imagine. The bewildered woman reluctantly makes a list. 'Well, it's worse than that,' the professional announces. 'Your child has got Down's syndrome.'

(The *Guardian*, Society, 23 October 2002, p. 11)

From any perspective, this example illustrates appalling practice. Bill had no such experiences, although his communications and interactions still had to be negotiated (and socially constructed?) with a variety of health care workers. He found the consultant very empowering.

Bill told the consultant during one visit that he always felt apprehensive (not frightened) when he came to the clinic. The doctor said that he need not, as he was unlikely to tell him anything that he did not already know himself. This was very empowering.

Sharing the news: Bill was not a medic and he did not 'need' to know about all the details of his disease/illness. The consultant treated him as an intelligent person, but this did not mean Bill was consulted as a medical colleague.

Bill was aware that most of the information transmitted during consultations was forgotten (or blocked). He kept a 'log', which helped him to feel 'grounded'. His friend also accompanied him and checked out the information.

Valiant efforts were made in the clinic to generate open communication systems: the names and functions of staff were posted; open evenings were held; leaflets were distributed and various groups were organised.

8 INCAPACITY BENEFITS

Bill was caught up in new rules, which were more stringent in relation to benefits.

He was given a sick note for the first five or six weeks of his early consultations and tests.

He was then expected to return to work.

He was given another sick note to cover the five weeks of radiotherapy.

His employers agreed to release him and to continue to pay his salary, although Bill was disappointed that the lack of a sick note meant the firm lost their contributions.

The GP told Bill that he did not seem the type to 'try it on'. (There was a new set of regulations for GPs.)

Bill had never been in this situation before; his GPs were very good but he still had to negotiate the deserving/undeserving issue.

9 PITCH YOUR TENT FOR ANOTHER NIGHT

The consultant had a sense of humour and invariably ended the session on a positive note. Clinics are not always 'doom and gloom' because for many patients they are (temporarily) cured or their vicissitudes are eased, even when they are dying. Bill made friends with other patients in the clinic; perhaps they belonged to the 'fellowship of suffering'. This did not mean that they were morbidly preoccupied by their illness situations but that they shared their common interests, and were thankful for each new day.

REFERENCES

Coelho, G. V., Hamburg, D. A. and Adams, J. E. (eds) (1974) *Coping and Adaptation*, New York, Basic Books.

Moos, R. H. and Tsu, V. D. (1977) *Coping with Physical Illness*, New York, Plenum Medical.

Stanton, A. H. and Schwartz, S. (1954) *The Mental Hospital: A Study of Institutional Participation in Psychiatric Illness and Treatment*, London, Tavistock.

EIGHTEEN

MOMENTS IN TIME

Edited by Ann Brechin

A MOMENT IN TIME – 1

It is time for a cup of tea in the lounge of a residential care home for people with dementia. About twelve people share this part of the home and six are in the lounge at this moment. Janice is sleeping in an armchair and wakes to hear her neighbour being offered a cup of tea. 'Cup of tea for you, Dora?'

'Where's my tea, then? Why am I not getting any tea?' Janice demands. Janice angers quickly and seems to see the world as set against her. Her instant response is angry and complaining and is very characteristic. I look round (visiting my father at the other side of the room) feeling for the staff and feeling in myself the slightly irritated desire to rebuke her for her petulance. 'Here is your tea, Janice,' I instinctively want to say. 'Why do you think we would have forgotten you? You were asleep!'

Instead the male volunteer carer, Jim, who is nearest her, responds with delight to her waking. 'Hello, Janice,' he says warmly. 'Have you woken up now?' He crouches down by her chair, smiling at her.

'Hello,' she says.

'Have you had a nice sleep? How are you feeling?' All said warmly with a smile of greeting and relaxed eye-contact.

'Hello' – she smiles and reaches out towards him – 'Give us a kiss!' She kisses his cheek – once and then again. 'Ooh you're nice' and she laughs in delight.

'Would you like a cup of tea, Janice?'

'Ooh, yes please.'

(Ann Brechin, course team member)

A MOMENT IN TIME – 2

Mina, Bill, Linda and myself were sitting in the staff room having our half-hour lunch break, when our manager, Cathy, stuck her head around the door. She looked around and seeing me said, 'Jen, you know what you were saying in supervision about needing to leave early tomorrow because your children's school is closing early for the heating to be fixed. Well I'm sorry but it's just not on after all. I've just checked the directive from senior management on phone cover, if you go early there'll be no back-up.' She turned to go.

Well I felt livid, that same morning she'd already agreed to me finishing early the next day, without mentioning any senior management directive. She had said that so long as I made the hours up it was OK. Now she was backtracking. Worse, supervision was supposed to be confidential wasn't it? She was in the habit of saying unpleasant or difficult things on her way out or when there wasn't much time to challenge or discuss it. Practically, I hadn't made other arrangements for my children, and time to do it was now getting short. Confused, and caught off balance, I was getting up to say 'Now you just hang on a minute I've had enough of you forever changing your mind' ... when Mina, who shares an office with me, intervened.

'Cathy,' she said, standing up and smiling, 'I think Jen would like to talk to you about this privately, perhaps she could come and see you after we have finished lunch at one-thirty for ten minutes?' The others nodded (we're all fed up with these 'on the run' communications). Faced with the whole team Cathy agreed. By this time, I had taken a few deep breaths! 'Yes,' I said slowly, 'I would welcome that, as it's very difficult for me to change my plans now. Perhaps we can talk about finding someone else to cover the phones, in return for me covering for them another day.'

When I thought about this later, I was so glad that Mina had learned the art of buying time and stopped me jumping in to challenge in a clumsy and angry way. She is really skilled at choosing the right place and time to say things, unlike our team leader. She is usually calm and unhurried so that you really hear what she says and feel there is time to respond. She makes you feel that she is really interested in you.

Stepping back from it further afterwards there were other skills to identify. First Mina is a leveller in the team. She doesn't take sides but is able to see things from different points of view. She has a capacity to stand back, contain things, and then quite quickly frame words that make it possible to find a way through. She is also able to challenge assertively without becoming heated or embarrassed. She was so calm in managing something quite difficult in a constructive way.

Mina told me that she always used to find such situations difficult. Partly because she had been the middle child in a family of five and always seemed 'caught in the middle'. She had, though, been able to use this experience to have empathy for others, but had learned the skills of standing back and re-framing the situation on an assertiveness training for women course.

Later, the team were able to talk with Cathy in a team meeting about her habit of saying difficult things on her way out, or in a situation where it was difficult to follow the matter through with her. The team had identified something through Mina that we wished to build on. Cathy shared that she was isolated as the manager and that it could feel that the whole team were 'as one' in opposing her. Bill responded to this by saying that if the team could share some of the decision-making process, then some things wouldn't be problems. For example, he was in a position to cover for me on the duty rota, but hadn't known it was needed. So he did that and later I helped him out when he had to take time out for an appointment with his dentist.

(Course team member)

A MOMENT IN TIME – 3

It was a long train journey and people, like me, were withdrawing into sleep or books. Just gradually I became aware of a grandmother and her young granddaughter across the aisle. What caught me was the communication and the total absorption of each with the other. So often we are distracted by other concerns and demands outside the moment. This grandmother was totally engaged. She was listening and responding, following the interests and inclinations of the child, responding to her questions. They were drawing together and discussing the results earnestly. She was following her pointing finger at cows in fields and scarecrows. The granddaughter loved it. I found it spellbinding, this relaxed enjoyment of each other's attention.

(Adapted account from a developmental tester)

A MOMENT IN TIME – 4

I was really struck by a lecture I went to once. It was just an academic lecture, nothing particularly unusual, at a conference and with quite a big audience. But it really stayed with me somehow. The lecturer was so good. I can remember even now some of what was said. But the main thing that was so powerful was the way he spoke. It was so clear and so easy to grasp and he spoke in a way that just communicated itself to the audience. Everything was well prepared and thought through and he was there not to show off his knowledge but to communicate. He held the audience spellbound. The delivery was clear, concise and wonderfully interesting. During questions afterwards, even if people's questions weren't that clear, he somehow handled them with clarity and a deep respect for grasping what lay behind the questions.

(Adapted account from a developmental tester)

A MOMENT IN TIME – 5

I am at a funeral of a white woman – a long-time exile from the then apartheid South Africa. Many of her mourners are black and have known her as a deeply committed ally in the fight against apartheid as well as a mother of young children and close friend. The funeral service is very moving.

At one point a friend is reading a eulogy, telling the story of this amazing woman who had won their hearts and their trust. She begins to cry and cannot go on. Into that painful silence, as we share her sadness and her struggle to regain control, floats gently the most beautiful African song. Started by one woman, it is taken up by others and fills the air with a message of sisterhood and support.

The speaker lifts her head and smiles her gratitude through her tears. It gives her time and conveys acceptance of her grief. Instead of painful silence we have a wonderful moment of extraordinary communication.

(Course team member)

A MOMENT IN TIME – 6

My father's Alzheimer's was very advanced. He barely knew his family, needed support in everything from my mother and seldom now was able to string words together to make any sense. Within a few weeks he would be going into care and would die a year later. Part of the pain of all this for me was knowing that I had never resolved the difficult relationship we had had. Although I knew he had loved me, his criticisms and readiness to anger had led to an emotional separation on my part in order to protect myself. Now, I felt, it was too late. I would never be able to have the conversations I needed to have with him in order to feel properly reconciled.

On this particular day, he had been distressed, angry and tearful briefly over a hurt finger and in this emotional state was just settling down with lots of reassurance and a cup of tea. Quite out of the blue, he looked at me across the room seeming to look deep into my eyes. I felt transfixed and very aware of real contact with my father. Time seemed to stand still as he spoke emotionally and falteringly. 'I wish,' he said, 'I wish . . . I could have . . . loved . . . better.'

The best I could do was to hold his gaze. I was completely incapable of responding in any other way, although I was profoundly moved.

I was left with a sense of failure that I had been so unable to respond – why couldn't I have said something, or simply moved to kiss him or hold his hand to show him I understood and how much I appreciated what he had said? It took yet another moment in time before I was able to find a positive way of coping with this memory.

Some time after my father had died I was talking to my daughter on the phone and found myself explaining the deep regret I felt that I had failed somehow to complete the exchange. He had offered me that – and I had done nothing at all in response.

'Perhaps you didn't need to', she said. 'Perhaps that was his gift to you. All you had to do was to receive it.'

That simple communication made such a difference to how I felt.

(Course team member)

A MOMENT IN TIME – 7

I am in a role-play. I am playing a senior staff nurse on a psychiatric ward where we have instigated a monthly review meeting where difficult cases are presented for discussion. The psychiatrist attends and (played in fact by a psychiatrist) is grandiose, patronising, overbearing, rather dismissive and completely unhelpful.

We role-play for a bit – I am gamely trying to chair the meeting and support the colleague whose case is under discussion. We break for discussion. The challenge to us all is to think what could we do to work successfully with this man. Various suggestions are made, featuring, not surprisingly, attempts to get the better of him, to teach him a lesson, to belittle him in turn. But our challenge is to 'find a way of being loving towards him'. What can we do that might actually make him feel appreciated and perhaps in turn enhance his capacity to help us?

I am working hard on myself at this point, trying to stem my irritation with this character we have jointly created. And I suddenly get there. What I find is an explanation that makes sense of his behaviour – an interpretation that is kind to him. And as soon as I begin to sense what is discomfiting him I can see a way forward. So I throw my suggestion into the ring with the others and am subsequently asked to role-play it out with the group again.

What I do is to suggest that I feel the discussion group had been a good idea but that I don't feel we have got the format right yet. I wonder if we could perhaps agree to spend a bit of time going back to basic principles and thinking about how we could improve matters. With everyone's agreement, we then discuss some of the ground rules. I say that I feel as if the group dynamic somehow always turns things around as if we are setting up Dr X by expecting him to come out with the answers, which I'm sure is not really a comfortable position to put him in. The dynamic of the role-play is extraordinary in that his demeanour changes totally as he agrees with obvious relief. We can then go on to explore how best we can draw in the group on the kind of input that it would be comfortable for people to make.

The workshop was called 'Enjoying the company of impossible people'. It was a powerful learning experience for me and I have used this role-play experience many times since as a reference point for myself. I realised that this willingness to accept someone, whose qualities aren't the ones you intuitively like, isn't so easy to develop. First comes the ability to deal with your own inner discomfort, and also to sense from that the discomfort of others. Then there is the need to resist the opportunity for revenge or for putting someone down, when for a moment those in power are in your power.

(Course team member)

NINETEEN

EXTERNALIZING THE PROBLEM

Michael White and David Epston

'Externalizing' is an approach to therapy that encourages persons to objec-
tify and, at times, to personify the problems that they experience as
oppressive. In this process, the problem becomes a separate entity and thus
external to the person or relationship that was ascribed as the problem.
Those problems that are considered to be inherent, as well as those relatively fixed qualities that are attributed to persons and to relationships, are
rendered less fixed and less restricting.

I (M. W.) began my first systematic attempts at encouraging persons to
externalize their problems approximately ten years ago. These attempts
took place predominantly within the context of work with families that
presented for therapy with problems identified in children.
[. . .]

The externalization of the child's problem clearly had great appeal for
these families. Although the problem was usually defined as internal to the
child, all family members were affected and often felt overwhelmed, dispir-
ited and defeated. In various ways, they took the ongoing existence of the
problem and their failed attempts to solve it as a reflection on themselves,
each other, and/or their relationships. The continuing survival of the
problem and the failure of corrective measures served to confirm, for
family members, the presence of various negative personal and relationship
qualities or attributes. Thus, when the members of these families detailed
the problems for which they were seeking therapy, it was not at all
unusual for them to present what I call a 'problem-saturated description'
of family life.
[. . .]

Source: White, M, Epston D. *Narrative Means to Therapeutic Ends*. New York (NY):
WW Norton & Co., Inc., 1990.

The very positive responses to . . . early systematic attempts at encouraging families to externalize their problems led me to extend this practice to a wide range of presenting problems. Throughout my subsequent explorations of this approach, I have found the externalization of the problem to be helpful to persons in their struggle with problems. Consequently, I have concluded that, among other things, this practice:

1   Decreases unproductive conflict between persons, including those disputes over who is responsible for the problem;
2   Undermines the sense of failure that has developed for many persons in response to the continuing existence of the problem despite their attempts to resolve it;
3   Paves the way for persons to cooperate with each other, to unite in a struggle against the problem, and to escape its influence in their lives and relationships;
4   Opens up new possibilities for persons to take action to retrieve their lives and relationships from the problem and its influence;
5   Frees persons to take a lighter, more effective, and less stressed approach to 'deadly serious' problems; and
6   Presents options for dialogue, rather than monologue, about the problem.

Within the context of the practices associated with the externalizing of problems, neither the person nor the relationship between persons is the problem. Rather, the problem becomes the problem, and then the person's relationship with the problem becomes the problem.

[. . .] Not only do the stories that persons have about their lives determine the meaning that they ascribe to experience, but these stories also determine which aspects of lived experience are selected out for the ascription of meaning. As Bruner (1986) argues, it is not possible for narratives to encompass the full richness of our lived experience:

> . . . *life experience is richer than discourse. Narrative structures organize and give meaning to experience, but there are always feelings and lived experience not fully encompassed by the dominant story.*
>
> (p. 143)

Since the stories that persons have about their lives determine both the ascription of meaning to experience and the selection of those aspects of experience that are to be given expression, these stories are constitutive or shaping of persons' lives. The lives and relationships of persons evolve as they live through or perform these stories.

Through the lens of the text analogy, various assumptions can be made about persons' experience of problems. Here I make the general assumption that, when persons experience problems for which they seek therapy, (a) the narratives in which they are storying their experience and/or in which they are having their experience storied by others do not sufficiently represent their lived experience, and (b), in these circumstances, there will be significant and vital aspects of their lived experience that contradict these dominant narratives.

The externalizing of the problem enables persons to separate from the dominant stories that have been shaping their lives and relationships. In so doing, persons are able to identify previously neglected but vital aspects of lived experience – aspects that could not have been predicted from a reading of the dominant story. Thus, following Goffman (1961), I have referred to these aspects of experience as 'unique outcomes' (White, 1987, 1988).

As unique outcomes are identified, persons can be encouraged to engage in performances of new meaning in relation to these. Success with this requires that the unique outcome be plotted into an alternative story about the person's life. I have referred to this alternative story as a 'unique account' and have developed an approach to questioning that encourages persons to locate, generate, or resurrect alternative stories that will 'make sense' of the unique outcomes.

[. . .]

RELATIVE INFLUENCE QUESTIONING

A general interviewing process that I have referred to as 'relative influence questioning' (White, 1986) is particularly effective in assisting persons to externalize the problem. This process of questioning is initiated at the outset of the first interview, so that persons are immediately engaged in the activity of separating their lives and relationships from the problem.

Relative influence questioning is comprised of two sets of questions. The first set encourages persons to map the influence of the problem in their lives and relationships. The second set encourages persons to map their own influence in the 'life' of the problem. By inviting persons to review the effects of the problem in their lives and relationships, relative influence questions assist them to become aware of and to describe their relationship with the problem. This takes them out of a fixed and static world, a world of problems that are intrinsic to persons and relationships, and into a world of experience, a world of flux. In this world, persons find new possibilities for affirmative action, new opportunities to act flexibly.

MAPPING THE INFLUENCE OF THE PROBLEM

Questions are introduced that encourage persons to map the influence of the problem in their lives and relationships. These questions assist persons to identify the problem's sphere of influence in the behavioural, emotional, physical, interactional, and attitudinal domains.

This involves a problem-saturated description of family life, which is much broader than the description that is usually offered of the problem 'itself'. Rather than restrict the investigation to the relationship between the problem and the person ascribed the problem, these questions identify the effect of the problem across various interfaces – between the problem and various persons, and between the problem and various relationships. This opens up a very broad field for the later search for unique outcomes and for the possibilities of affirmative action. Affirmative action might be taken across any of these interfaces. This makes it possible for all of those associated with the problem to experience a new sense of personal agency.

To illustrate the practice of 'mapping the influence of the problem', I have selected the problem of encopresis.

Nick, aged six years, was brought to see me by his parents, Sue and Ron. Nick had a very long history of encopresis, which had resisted all attempts to resolve it, including those instituted by various therapists. Rarely did a day go by without an 'accident' or 'incident', which usually meant the 'full works' in his underwear.

To make matters worse, Nick had befriended the 'poo'. The poo had become his playmate. He would 'streak' it down walls, smear it in drawers, roll it into balls and flick it behind cupboards and wardrobes, and had even taken to plastering it under the kitchen table. In addition, it was not uncommon for Ron and Sue to find soiled clothes that had been hidden in different locations around the house, and to discover poo pushed into various corners and squeezed into the shower and sink drains. The poo had even developed the habit of accompanying Nick in the bath.

In response to my questions about the influence of the poo in the lives and relationships of family members, we discovered that:

1   The poo was making a mess of Nick's life by isolating him from other children and by interfering with his school work. By coating his life, the poo was taking the shine off his future and was making it impossible for him and others to see what he was really like as a person. For example, this coating of poo dulled the picture of him as a person, making it difficult for other people to see what an interesting and intelligent person he was.
2   The poo was driving Sue into misery, forcing her to question her capacity to be a good parent and her general capability as a person. It was overwhelming her to the extent that she felt quite desperate and on the

verge of 'giving up'. She believed her future as a parent to be clouded with despair.

3   The ongoing intransigence of the poo was deeply embarrassing to Ron. This embarrassment had the effect of isolating him from friends and relatives. It wasn't the sort of problem that he could feel comfortable talking about to workmates. Also, the family lived in a relatively distant and small farming community, and visits of friends and relatives usually required that they stay overnight. These overnight stays had become a tradition. As Nick's 'accidents' and 'incidents' were so likely to feature in any such stay, Ron felt constrained in the pursuit of this tradition. Ron had always regarded himself as an open person, and it was difficult for him to share his thoughts and feelings with others and at the same time keep the 'terrible' secret.

4   The poo was affecting all the relationships in the family in various ways. For example, it was wedged between Nick and his parents. The relationship between him and Sue had become somewhat stressed, and much of the fun had been driven out of it. And the relationship between Nick and Ron had suffered considerably under the reign of tyranny perpetrated by the poo. Also, since their frustrations with Nick's problems always took center stage in their discussions, the poo had been highly influential in the relationship between Sue and Ron, making it difficult for them to focus their attention on each other.

MAPPING THE INFLUENCE OF PERSONS

Once a description of the problem's sphere of influence has been derived by mapping its effects in persons' lives and relationships, a second set of questions can be introduced. This set features those questions that invite persons to map their influence and the influence of their relationships in the 'life' of the problem. These questions bring forth information that contradicts the problem-saturated description of family life and assist persons in identifying their competence and resourcefulness in the face of adversity. [. . .]

After identifying Nick's, Sue's, and Ron's influence in the life of [what we came to call] Sneaky Poo, I introduced questions that encouraged them to perform meaning in relation to these examples, so that they might 're-author' their lives and relationships.

How had they managed to be effective against the problem in this way? How did this reflect on them as people and on their relationships? What personal and relationship attributes were they relying on in these achievements? Did this success give them any ideas about further steps that they might take to reclaim their lives from the problem? What difference would knowing what they now knew about themselves make to their future relationship with the problem?

In response to these questions, Nick thought that he was ready to stop Sneaky Poo from outsmarting him so much, and decided that he would not be tricked into being its playmate anymore. Sue had some new ideas for refusing to let Sneaky Poo push her into misery, and Ron thought that he just might be ready to take a risk and follow up with his idea of telling a workmate of his struggle with Sneaky Poo.

I met with this family again two weeks later. In that time Nick had had only one minor accident – this described as light 'smudging'. Sneaky Poo had tried to win him back after nine days, but Nick had not given in. He had taught Sneaky Poo a lesson – he would not let it mess up his life anymore. He described how he had refused to be tricked into playing with Sneaky Poo and believed that his life was no longer coated with it, that he was now shining through. He was talkative, happier, felt stronger, and was more physically active. Sneaky Poo had been a tricky character, and Nick had done very well to get his life back for himself.

Sue and Ron had also 'gotten serious' in their decision not to cooperate with the requirements of Sneaky Poo. Sue had started to 'treat herself' more often, particularly on those occasions during which Sneaky Poo was giving her a hard time, and 'had put her foot down', showing that it couldn't take her so lightly anymore.

Ron had taken a risk and had protested Sneaky Poo's isolation of him. He had talked to a couple of his workmates about the problem. They had listened respectfully, offering a few comments. An hour later, one of them had returned and had disclosed that he had been experiencing a similar problem with a son. There ensued a very significant conversation and a strengthening bond of friendship. And without that coating on Nick's life, Ron had discovered that 'Nick was good to talk to.'

I encouraged Nick, Sue, and Ron to reflect on and speculate about what this success said about the qualities that they possessed as people and about the attributes of their relationships. I also encouraged them to review what these facts suggested about their current relationship with Sneaky Poo. In this discussion, family members identified further measures that they could take to decline Sneaky Poo's invitations to support it.

We met on a third occasion three weeks later, and I discovered that all had proceeded to take further steps to outrun Sneaky Poo, steps to ensure that it would be put in its proper place. Nick had made some new friends and had been catching up on his school work, and the family had visited overnight with several friends and relatives. Sue was making good her escape from guilt. This had been facilitated, to an extent, by the fact that she and Ron had been talking more to other parents about the trials and tribulations of parenting. In so doing they had learned that they were not the only parents who had doubts about their parenting skills.

We then did some contingency planning, just in case Sneaky Poo tried to make a comeback and to outstreak Nick again. I saw this family again one month later for a review. At the six-month follow-up, Nick was doing very well. Only on one or two occasions had there been a slight smudging on his pants. He was more confident and doing even better with friends and at school. Everyone felt happy with his progress.

DEFINING THE PROBLEM TO BE EXTERNALIZED

In the practices associated with externalizing the problem, care is taken to ensure that the person's description of it and of its effects in their lives and relationships are privileged.
[. . .]
As with any approach to working with persons who seek therapy, it is important that therapists do make generalizations about situations, but keep in mind the specifics of every circumstance and think ahead to the likely consequences of particular courses of action. This argues for a certain level of 'consciousness' on the therapist's behalf. Further, lest the therapist inadvertently contribute to persons' experiences of oppressions, this consciousness requires an appreciation of local politics – that is, politics at the level of relationships. [. . .]

REFERENCES

Bruner, E. (1986) 'Ethnography as narrative', in V. Turner and E. Bruner (eds) *The Anthology of Experience*, Chicago, University of Illinois Press.

Goffman, E. (1961) *Asylums: Essays in the Social Situation of Mental Patients and Other Inmates*, New York, Doubleday.

White, M. (1986) 'Negative explanation, restraint and double description: a template for family therapy', *Family Process*, Vol. 25, No. 2.

White, M. (1987) 'Family therapy and schizophrenia: addressing the "In-the-corner lifestyle" ', *Dulwich Centre Newsletter*, Spring.

White, M. (1988) 'The process of questioning: a therapy of literary merit?', *Dulwich Centre Newsletter*, Winter.

TWENTY

COUNSELLING FOR TOADS

Robert de Board

TOAD'S FIRST MEETING WITH HIS COUNSELLOR

It would take too long to narrate all that happened over the next few days. First Toad was nursed by his friends. Then they encouraged him. Then they told him, quite sternly, to pull himself together. Finally, they spelled out the drab and dismal future facing him unless he 'got a grip of himself', as Badger eloquently put it.

But none of this had any effect on Toad. He responded as best he could, but there were no signs of the old Toad, full of life and eager to outwit their well-meant exhortations. Instead he remained sad and depressed, and the more his friends advised him in detail what he should do, the more sad and depressed he became.

Finally, Badger could stand it no longer. That admirable animal, though long on exhortation, was short on patience.

'Now, look here Toad, this can go on no longer. We are all trying to help you, but it seems you won't (or can't, thought Mole perceptively) help yourself. There is only one thing left. You must have counselling!'

There was a shocked silence. Even Toad sat up a little straighter. None of the animals knew fully what counselling meant, but they knew it was a mysterious activity undertaken by people who had experienced some severe or shocking event. The Rat, who was a traditionalist at heart, said, 'Do you really think Toad is that bad? I mean, don't you think it's a bit

Source: de Board, R. *Counselling for Toads*. London: Routledge, 1998.
Reproduced by permission.

trendy, all this counselling? It seems from the newspapers that everyone these days is given counselling. In my day, people in trouble were given a couple of aspirin. It probably did them more good.' Ratty remembered that the original suggestion about counselling had come from him and he was beginning to get cold feet.

'But we've got the address of a local counsellor,' said the Mole. 'I thought we had agreed that Toad ought to see him. I agree with Badger.'

'Well said, Mole,' answered Badger. 'You mustn't be worried, Ratty. Toad must be in a very poor state of health if even the advice I can offer appears to fall on deaf ears. I know that you can be obstinate, Toad, but it does seem that you need some kind of help which, surprisingly, your friends cannot give you. Desperate circumstances require desperate remedies. We must try counselling.'

And so it happened that, after much telephoning and arranging and pushing and pleading, Toad arrived at a large house called The Heronry. It was a foursquare three-storeyed building of red brick mellowed to a terracotta colour with occasional bands of yellow. It had an air of permanence and sensible values and looked the sort of house where a family might remain for a long time. After ringing the bell, Toad was shown to a book-lined room with some chairs and a large desk on which sat odds and ends, including a china head with words written all over the skull. It bore the legend 'Phrenology by L. N. Fowler'. The Heron entered, looking tall and wise, and sat on the chair opposite Toad. He wished Toad good morning and then sat quietly looking at him. Toad, who had become used to people talking at him, waited for the lecture to begin. But nothing happened. In this silence, Toad could feel the blood pulsing in his head and it seemed as if this was pumping up the tension in the room. He began to feel very uncomfortable. The Heron continued to look at him. Finally Toad could stand it no longer.

'Aren't you going to tell me what to do?' he asked plaintively.

'About what?' answered Heron.

'Well, tell me what I have to do to get better.'

'Are you feeling unwell?'

'Yes I am. But surely they have told you all about me?'

'Who are "they"?' asked Heron.

'Oh, you know. Badger and Rat and all that lot.' And with those words Toad started to cry and let loose a flood of unhappiness that, all unknowingly, he had kept pent up for a long time. The Heron remained silent but pushed a box of tissues nearer to him. Eventually Toad's sobs subsided and he drew breath, and he felt a little better. Then the Heron spoke.

'Would you like to tell me why you are here?'

'I am here', said Toad, 'because they made me come. They said that I needed counselling and they got your name from the newspaper. And I am ready to listen to you and do whatever you think best. I know that they have my best interests at heart.'

The Counsellor shifted in his chair. 'So who is my client, you or them?'
Toad did not quite understand.

'Look,' said the Counsellor, 'your friends want me to counsel you so
that their worry about you will be relieved. You seem to want to be helped
in order to please them. So I think that my client is really your friends.'
Toad was confused by all this and clearly showed it.

'Perhaps we can clarify the situation,' said the Counsellor. 'Who is
going to pay for these meetings?'

I might have guessed, thought Toad. He's just like the rest of them, only
anxious about getting paid.

'You don't need to worry about that,' said Toad, feeling a little like his
old self. 'Badger said he would take care of the money side of things. You
will get paid, never fear.'

'Thank you,' said the Counsellor, 'but I am afraid that this won't do at
all. I suggest that we conclude this meeting and put it down to experience.'

For the first time in many days, Toad began to feel angry. 'Look here,'
he said in a stronger voice, 'you can't do that. You call yourself a counsellor and I have come here for counselling. I have sat here waiting for you to
tell me something and now all you can say is that my money isn't good
enough. What more do I have to do to get things started?'

'That is a very good question and I will answer it,' the Counsellor
responded. 'Counselling is always a voluntary process, both for the counsellor and for the client. That means we can only work together if you
want to do this for your own sake and not just to please your friends. If
we agree to work together we need to make a contact, and then, at the
completion of our work, I would send my invoice to you. You see, it's not
a question of money. But this can only be your responsibility and no one
else's.'

Toad's mind was racing. Without understanding the full import of the
words, he realised that somehow he was being asked to take responsibility
for his own counselling. And yet he was not the counsellor!

At the same time, the Counsellor had used the word 'work' and this
implied Toad's active involvement in whatever might happen. All this was
a long way from his initial attitude of waiting for somebody to tell him
what to do. These thoughts were disturbing but at the same time, exciting.
Maybe there was a way out of his misery which he could discover for
himself. After what seemed an age, Toad spoke.

'I seem to have made rather an ass of myself and not for the first time.
But I think I am beginning to see what you are getting at and I would like
to work with you. Can we start again?'

'I rather think that we have started already,' replied the Counsellor. He
then went on to spell out in detail what it would mean if they agreed to
work together on a counselling programme.

'We would meet together for an hour once a week, for as long as
required. I suggest every Tuesday at ten in the morning, starting next

week. At the final session we will review what we have done and what you have learnt and you can consider any future plans you may wish to make.'

'And how much do you charge?' asked the practical Toad.

'Forty pounds per session,' replied Heron. 'I will invoice you for that amount at the completion of each session.' Then after a considerable pause he added, 'Well have you decided what you would like to do?'

Toad did not often make considered decisions. Either he made them on the spur of the moment and lived to regret it, like driving off in a motorcar which just happened to take his fancy, or else he did what he was told, usually by Badger, and felt miserable as a result. He would have liked to have asked the sensible Rat, 'Ratty, what do you think I should do?' and have the responsibility taken from his shoulders. But the Heron was looking at him in a particular way as if he was quite certain that he, Toad, would make a sensible decision. He finally said, 'I would like to work with you and try to discover why I am feeling so miserable and what I can do to improve things. I have got my diary here. Shall we agree on those dates?'

As the Counsellor was seeing Toad to the door, Toad turned to him and said, 'Do you think that there is some hope for me of getting better?'

The Heron stopped and looked him straight in the eye. 'Toad, if I did not think that we are all capable of change and improvement, I would not be doing this work. It is not inevitable that things get better. But what I can promise is that you will have my full and undivided attention. And I shall expect the same commitment from you. If we both work together like that then we can expect a positive outcome. However, in the last analysis, it all depends on you.'

Toad walked down the path, trying to understand what those words meant.

[. . .]

THE NEXT MEETING

Toad met the Counsellor the following week and sat in his usual seat. He was surprised how quickly he was getting used to the routine and he now thought of the chair as 'his' chair. Sometimes he wondered if anyone else ever sat in it, or if the room was only used once a week for him.

But the thing that impressed him most about these counselling sessions was receiving the Heron's full and undivided attention. Toad began to realise that he had never before received anyone's full attention in his entire life. Whether he had ever given it to anyone was a question yet to be asked.

The Heron listened to him attentively all the time. It was as if, for an hour, he centred himself entirely on Toad and focused on his situation to the exclusion of all else. Consequently, he found that he did not have to keep saying, 'Do you see what I mean?' or 'Have I made myself clear?', which he habitually found himself using to excuse his waffle and imprecision.

Providing that he, Toad, found the words to describe what he was thinking, the Heron listened and understood. But when he failed to understand, he would say so and then Toad would be forced to be more precise and search for other words and expressions which would convey his meaning more exactly.

Somehow, the way in which the Heron listened to him and prodded him with questions enabled him to bring all sorts of thoughts and feelings to consciousness. Gradually he was beginning to explore and examine aspects of himself of which previously he had been unaware. In other words, Toad had started to learn.

'Well Toad,' said the Heron. 'How are you feeling?' This question no longer surprised him and in fact he was expecting it.

'I'm feeling different,' he answered. 'I'm still low in my spirits, but I keep finding myself thinking about our previous meeting, when you talked about Child Ego State. Are we going to talk about it any more this time?'

'Yes,' said the Heron. 'I would like to explore that with you. But it means that I must change roles.'

'What do you mean?' asked Toad.

'It means', replied the Heron, 'that I shall behave differently. If I am to teach you about the Child State, I must take on the role of the teacher. One of the differences will be that I shall be in a telling mode, rather than a listening mode. If I successfully teach you about the Child Ego State, then you will be able to use those ideas to explore your own self and your own experience. Remember, there is nothing so practical as a good theory!'

As Toad was trying to puzzle out just what that meant, the Heron stood up and went to the flip-chart.

'The Child Ego State', he began, 'is made up of the archaic relics of our childhood. It consists of all the emotions we experienced when we were little. You must remember that at birth, we start out with only the very basic emotions. In our early years, these gradually develop into more subtle and complex patterns of behaviour which become central to our very self and form part of us, defining our behaviour for the rest of our lives. The result is that now, in particular situations and circumstances which are different for each of us, we respond automatically from that basic position. Once again, we act and feel like the child we once were.'

'Could you explain that a bit more, please?' asked Toad.

'Certainly,' replied the Heron. 'I am suggesting that we are born with certain basic emotions, rather like the primary colours, which are similar for all babies. But as we develop as individuals, our feelings and responses become increasingly individualistic, just as basic colours mix together to create all sorts of subtle shades and hues. Does that make sense?'

'Yes,' said Toad, 'I can understand that.'

'Right then,' answered the Heron. 'What do you think these basic emotions are?' Toad frowned and scratched his head, but was unable to come up with the answer.

'Look at it this way,' said the Heron. 'I know you are not married, but do you have any nephews or nieces?'

'Yes of course,' said the Toad, 'I always remember their birthdays and I love taking them their presents at Christmas. In fact, I think they're rather fond of me.'

'Good,' replied the Heron. 'So how would you define some of their basic emotions?'

'Well they are usually rushing about all over the place, having fun. I don't know where they get all that energy! And then when I arrive, all laden with presents, they throw themselves at me and give me the most tremendous kisses and hugs. Very cheering, really. Mind you,' continued Toad, 'it's not just the presents. I get the same kind of welcome whenever I go. They're just very affectionate.'

'I'm sure they are,' said Heron. 'Let's write this up.' So he went to the flip-chart and wrote the heading 'Children's Basic Emotions' and underneath, 'Fun and Affection'.

'Any others?' the Heron asked.

'They can certainly get angry with each other,' said Toad. 'I've known them have the most terrible fights when I have had to separate them physically. They can be little devils.'

'So there's another basic emotion,' said Heron, and wrote 'Anger' on the chart.

'Oh yes,' said the Toad, 'I certainly agree with that.'

'Can you think of any others?' asked Heron.

'I'm a bit stuck,' Toad replied, after a pause.

'Try thinking of it in another way,' said the Heron. 'What are the basic emotions we seem to be born with, which just come naturally, without having to be learnt?'

'I'm not sure if this is what you are after,' said Toad, 'but my little nephews and nieces can easily get upset and sad. I remember on my last visit, they were crying because their puppy had just died. I tried to comfort them, they were all in tears. But I wasn't much help. Ended up crying myself. I'm really very soft-hearted, you know.' Here Toad blew his nose and fiddled with his bow-tie and his eyes were bright with tears.

'That seems like a very basic emotion,' said the Heron and wrote 'Sadness' on the list. 'Any others?'

Toad shook his head. 'I can't think of one.'

'How about fear?' asked the Heron. 'In my experience, children can easily become scared and it's very easy to frighten a child. Unbelievably, some adults seem to enjoy doing just that, but that's another story. Anyhow, do you agree with fear?'

'Most certainly,' Toad replied. 'I can still remember waking up scream-ing from my first nightmare when I was very small. And no one taught me to behave like that. I just yelled. It came naturally.'

'Right,' said the Heron. 'So I think that completes our list,' and he added 'Fear' to it. So this was what was finally written on the flip-chart:

Children's Basic Emotions
Fun and Affection
Anger
Sadness
Fear

'All of these emotions added together make up what is called the "Natural Child" and this forms a significant part of the total Child Ego State,' said the Counsellor.

'So', said Toad, 'when I see someone being affectionate or getting angry or sad or frightened, I can say that they are in their Natural Child. Is that right?'

'Exactly,' said the Heron, 'although anger is more complex and we shall learn more about that particular emotion later on.'

'And people can be in their Child State no matter how old they are?' asked Toad.

'Most certainly,' replied the Heron. 'People get into their Child State and feel and act exactly the same as they did when they were little, quite irrespective of their chronological age.'

There was a long silence as Toad fell into deep thought. Finally he spoke.

'I think', he said, 'that I am often in the Child Ego State,' and lapsed back into silence.

'But', said Heron, 'that's only half the picture.'

'What do you mean?' said Toad. 'Is there more to be said about this Child Ego State?'

'There certainly is,' replied Heron. 'A great deal more. As we have seen, a child's natural behaviour is a mixture of these basic emotions,' and he pointed to the list on the flip-chart.

'For instance, a baby will scream for food and attention, drink as much milk as it can get and then sleep when it is replete and content. All those natural feelings come into operation from day one and as the baby grows physically stronger so its emotional life develops and becomes more powerful.

'But there are other factors which come into play. And the most import-ant of these is the baby's parents. They impinge on its consciousness right from the beginning. Almost everything the baby does causes some response from its mother or father and these have a profound influence on the child.

'Usually a mother responds to her baby's cry with love and comforting behaviour. But parents can act in an unloving way. The mother may be tired and even ill and respond harshly. Or the father may have strict views on how children should be reared and may deliberately ignore the baby's cries for fear of "spoiling" it.'

'It makes you realise just how vulnerable babies are,' Toad said thoughtfully. 'I never realised before just what power people have over their children. They have total dominion. They can love them or reject them, cuddle them or abuse them. It's just a lottery what sort of parents you get.'

He sat very quietly, thinking deeply about his own childhood, trying to remember what it felt like. After a while, the Heron spoke again.

'You're quite right, Toad,' he said. 'Most parents try to do their best and very few want anything but good for their children. But parents are only human and they inevitably pass on their beliefs and behaviours to their offspring as surely as they pass on their genes. And children just have to learn to cope and defend themselves from the consequences.'

'But how can they learn to cope?' asked Toad, now quite animated and obviously thinking hard. 'Babies and little children can't think logically. They can't sit down and plan how to cope with their mother's or father's behaviour.' He said this quite strongly, as if he was dealing, not with an abstruse point of child psychology, but with something deeply personal. As indeed he was.

'Well, of course a baby or an infant can't think through these issues logically or consciously,' said Heron. 'But what they do is to learn through experience. This kind of learning involves not just our brains but our total self. What we learn is a strategy for living. We develop behaviours which enable us to cope with our parents and others. And if we are lucky, we have enough energy left over to enjoy life.

'This means that every baby must learn how to adapt his or her basic behaviour to cope with their primal situation. These adaptations become the nucleus around which the rest of our behaviour grows and develops. Of course, we are influenced by many other events later in our lives. But these earliest experiences shape the beginning of us and we can never deny or forget them.'

'Could you slow down a bit?' pleaded Toad. 'Just when I think that I have grasped something, you go on to something else.'

'I'm sorry,' smiled the Heron. 'I know that I tend to go on a bit about this, but I believe it to be of the greatest importance. In all our work together, Toad, understanding your childhood is the key to understanding yourself. As Freud said, "Where there is Id, there shall Ego be." But I'll explain that later. Now Toad, what was it in particular that you did not understand?'

'You said that as we learn to cope with our lives as infants, we have to make 'adaptations' to our natural behaviour. What does that mean?'

'That's an excellent question,' answered Heron. 'Let me answer by telling you a short story. It's science fiction, so you can let your imagination run free.

'Imagine a small planet on which there are only three living beings, yourself and two others. These two other beings are more than twice your height and you are completely dependent on them for everything. This includes not only your food but also your emotional needs. Usually they treat you well and then you respond by loving them. But sometimes they get angry with you and this makes you feel frightened and unhappy. And because they are so big and powerful, you feel helpless. What do you think about that?'

'I don't much like that story,' answered Toad. 'If that was me, I would build a spaceship and escape from those two creatures as fast as I could.'

'Unfortunately, you can't escape. So you are just going to have to put up with the situation and learn how to cope as best you can.'

'In other words,' said Toad, who had caught on to the real meaning of the story, 'I shall have to learn to adapt my behaviour to this particular situation.'

'Well done,' replied Heron. 'You really are learning now. For as you have realised, my story is a parable of infancy. We start our lives with only two, or sometimes only one other person in our life. They are so much bigger than us and we are totally dependent on them. As there is no escape, our only option is to adapt to their every whim. Let me draw a simple diagram to illustrate this.'

He went to the flip-chart and drew a circle and wrote above it, 'The Child Ego State'. Then he divided the circle in half with a horizontal line. In the top half he wrote 'Natural Child'. In the bottom half he wrote 'Adapted Child'.

'Now Toad,' said Heron, 'we must finish here. It's been a very full session and I am sure it has given you a lot to think about. So let me give you some homework for our next meeting.'

'Oh no,' said Toad, looking quite anxious, 'not homework! I always hated doing prep. I don't think I shall be able to do any this week. In fact I've just remembered I have a lot of work to do. I will probably have to go up to town. And lots of other things,' he added lamely. There was a long silence.

'Just as a matter of interest,' said Heron, 'how would you analyse what you have just said to me?'

'Well,' said Toad, 'I simply told you why I am unable to do any homework.' He looked uneasy and found it difficult to meet Heron's eye.

'Yes, but how do you think it sounded to me?' Toad shifted in his chair. 'I don't know really. I merely gave you the reasons why I can't do it.'

'Were they reasons?' asked Heron. There was a long pause. Then Toad spoke.

'Perhaps you thought they sound like excuses?'

'What do you think?' asked Heron.

'I can understand you thinking that,' answered Toad, 'but the word "homework" gives me very bad feelings. I can remember exactly how I felt at school in the evenings trying to learn Latin verbs or memorise poetry. And then the fear of punishment the next morning if you got it wrong.'

'So what state were you in when I suggested homework to you just now?' asked Heron.

'Child,' replied Toad instantly. 'All those old fears and anxieties came sweeping over me. Is there something wrong with me, Heron, that I should behave like that?'

'No, of course not,' said Heron warmly. 'We all have words or situations which trigger off our childhood feelings. I suppose the most commonly shared word that can do this is "dentist".'

'Oh no, not the dentist!' said Toad, clutching his jaw in mock agony.

'So I will avoid the dreaded "homework" word,' said Heron, 'and instead ask you simply to do some work before our next meeting.'

'What kind of work?' asked Toad, still a little on the defensive.

'Just think about your own childhood. Think about those early days and your earliest memories. And then we can see if our work here throws any light on them. Goodbye Toad. I look forward to seeing you next week.'

TWENTY-ONE

'THE MEMORY BIRD': ACCOUNTS BY SURVIVORS OF SEXUAL ABUSE – EXTRACT 1

Brenda Nicklinson

EXPERIENCES OF THERAPY

I look back over all these years [of therapy] and see how much and how often I was disempowered and abused in various ways; how ethical issues sometimes became the tool for some kinds of abuse, how my trust was betrayed, how my being a victim was taken advantage of, how my therapy sometimes became therapy to heal the abuse of therapy, how concepts such as transference and projection were sometimes used to deny my reality: for example my seeing real damage happening in the present was said to be simply my transference feelings. So often, theories and concepts were used to enable the therapist to control me and as a wall to protect himself. I think, too, of how my paid-for time was often taken up by counter-transference issues that were not recognised. I think one of the most disempowering and constantly repeated abuses was the denial of my feelings, my truth, my process. Fragile and fractured though it was, it was always there trying to be heard.

When I look back and ask myself in what way and how much has therapy empowered me, I can say only inasmuch as I was respected and believed and listened to, only inasmuch as my process was accepted and worked with, only inasmuch as my reality was validated, only inasmuch as the exploration was a shared experience and not under someone else's

Source: Malone, C, Farthing, L, Marce, L. *The Memory Bird. Survivors of Sexual Abuse.* London: Virago Press, 1996. Reproduced by permission.

control, only inasmuch as there was safety, only inasmuch as there was a certain degree of flexibility and willingness to hear my story, only inasmuch as there was openness and honesty and genuineness and a meeting.

And the worst part of it all has been my vulnerability as a client, my having no one to turn to or support me, my having to try to do battle with or make things safe for therapists whilst totally alone, and my having to do that from the weaker position of client whilst in the midst of the distress caused by the various sorts of hurt and/or abuse, in order to try to protect myself. It has been horrific that the severe abuse that happened to me originally has been the cause of more abuse. It was terrible not to be heard, not to be believed. It was terrible to be encouraged to trust and then to have that trust betrayed, to trust and not be trusted. It was horrific to have my barriers broken down and then be hurt in ways that were beyond my capacity to take or protect myself from; being unable to protect myself or leave because my need to heal was so great.

And in the same way as I have been helped in therapy by those helping me believing and witnessing and supporting me, I have been helped by those who were able to believe and witness and support me when the therapeutic situation became damaging, especially if the therapist himself was able to take that on and admit the mistake and help me to work through the hurt.

TWENTY-TWO

DONNA

Donna

Society tells me I'm black – God tells me I'm a human being. Growing up as a black woman, having children and seeing what happened to other black people all showed me that white society has not cared for Black people. In 1995, I was at a time in my life when I felt pretty vulnerable and needing help, but yet also saw that this brought up complex issues about Black people and therapy. I was reluctant to get help from a (white) institution. But finally I contacted my (white) GP, although at first I was not sure what I was asking for. I was aware of the possible harmfulness of therapy for Black people – the medical model gives nothing. Also I would put myself in a vulnerable position with records on me. Desperate at the time, I would have done anything and would have gladly taken medication, but my GP recommended counselling. After I agreed, I agonised over my decision for weeks before my appointment was due. I was always aware that my counsellor would probably be white and middle class – Black people are under-represented in therapy. I never prayed so much in my life and asked the Creator that I got a counsellor who would not shut me down and who would help me deal with my problem effectively. I was willing to take a chance, as part of me was still aware of myself, my wants and needs.

As soon as I go in that room with the [white] therapist it's political as far as I'm concerned. At first I was worried that I could lose myself in that therapy – give my mind over to a white woman. So there was no way I was gonna get swallowed into anything ... until that power is not happening. At the beginning I talked about my therapy with my [black] woman friend. As time went on I began to raise particular issues with my counsellor and asked her perfect questions as to her own background and attitude to Black people and counselling. I also had to risk not holding how I felt back from

Source: Newnes, C. (ed.) *Changes*, vol. 18, no. 4 (Winter) 2000. Reproduced by permission.

her. It was a chance that I didn't really want to take because if she had to refer me on, then she was going to refer me to another white person. To take the risk I created a space for myself by gradually starting asking questions, and requesting to see particular notes on myself, which before doing a counselling course in 1993 I was not aware I was entitled to.

My therapist made me see things clearly – or she might trigger something off – and then I would go and do something else about it. But the main problem throughout was that I just didn't know where she was coming from. That was the problem for me. Didn't know what experiences she had had. I have had experiences of white people being very good at acting, and being so convincing sometimes. Not knowing where she was coming from didn't make me feel comfortable and made me hold back. Questions kept popping up in my head and needed asking so I tackled her about it on the sixth session by saying 'I'm just wasting my time coming here'. I wanted her to have a *little* understanding that it was not easy coming from where I'm coming. So I took the chance anyway and gave her the name of 'Isis Papers' (a book by Frances Cress-Welsing, 1991). I was looking to see if there would be a reaction in our next session. It was a breakthrough for me to see her in her position (of therapist) still being consistent because this is a POWERful book. That really uplifted me that. It was like I had to give her that space – that trust.

At times I struggled with the language. Even though we all speak English, I find that professionals and white people do not understand Black English – my language. That means that therapy and what I could benefit from can be blocked and nothing develops. I felt it was up to me to change my language to try to be understood. Sometimes I thought my therapist didn't really understand what I was saying or meaning and so I needed to check her out on it.

I am grateful that I didn't get 'shit' through being in counselling or that she did my head in more than what it was than when I came in. Because I needed to sort myself out: I've got things to do and she helped me a lot. Although I don't think my therapist understood what was going on for me from a black issue – I think she understands it from a human being's perspective because the pain and the suffering and all that what I have is no different to what you or her will have: but the situation's different.

For me the main thing that came out with the therapy and change for me was to work with my personal POWER more. That includes having a little more support – from anybody in my life. My therapist educated me as well, showing that there is room for change; that I don't have to just take things and say 'thank you'. Also I would say to therapists – if you have got the power, be responsible and use it properly.

REFERENCE

Cress-Welsing, F. (1991) *The Isis (Yssis) Papers*, Chicago, Third World Press.

TWENTY-THREE

TELLING OTHER PEOPLE

Edited by Ann Richardson and Dietmar Bolle

One of the first questions on being diagnosed [with AIDS or HIV] is who to tell. There can be very reassuring reactions.

IMRAT (MALAYSIA)

I went to Australia and, for the first three months there, I was losing weight and had diarrhoea and terrible flu. Two months after, I was still losing weight. The doctor put us [on] to another doctor, who said that we'll probably have to run an AIDS test.

In Malaysia at that time, AIDS did not exist, nobody talked about it. Of course, we heard about it in the papers, it's an epidemic hitting the US, but we had not had any cases or nobody knew about them. So the first thing I told the doctor, 'Look,' I said, 'as far as I'm concerned we Malaysians don't get AIDS.'

I went for the test, and one week after the results came back positive. The only knowledge I had at that time was if you have AIDS you die – you have no hopes. I was confused, depressed, really terrified. I said that's it, I probably have a month or two months to live.

I called my family. I told them I'm sick, I'm not feeling well and I probably have this thing called AIDS. The immediate reaction was – I'm the only son in the family – my brother-in-law flew down from Singapore. He didn't talk to me about being gay or having AIDS, he just ignored the whole topic. The main concern was to bring me back home.

He booked a flight the next day. It was quite depressing. I was crying all

Source: Richardson, A, Bolle, D. (eds) *Wise before Their Time*. London: HarperCollins, 1992. Reproduced by permission.

the way, trying to think how will I face my family. Because I knew that my whole family will be there, waiting for me to come back. I was not ashamed of what I had, it was more talking to them about it. They'd probably think that I did something sinful, something that's dirty. This is what I was afraid of, facing them.

I was really surprised when we came in the airport. My mum was there, my dad, my sisters, they all came and hugged me and they saw how weak I was. I think they had the same idea as I had – that I'm going to die.

PETER (USA)

It was difficult to tell my lover I had HIV. I did it on the very first trip that he came to visit, about six weeks after I'd found out. I had presumed that as soon as he knew, he would walk out. His reaction, after we had discussed it, was where would I walk *to*? It was very endearing, made us much closer, there's no question about that.

When I decided that I would tell, everybody was going to be told. I made no list. Because I knew that if I tell one person, that person may just run into another person and so on. If they are truly friends, they're entitled to my well-being and they're also entitled to my bad-being or my worst-being.

The one unfortunate part was that before I could tell my mother and sister, a friend of mine – former friend – decided to tell them instead. I had not counted on that happening. If I'm going to tell somebody that I'm HIV-positive, I want to tell them in person. When I see the reaction, I can cater to it. My sister phoned and said, 'Is this true?' and I said, 'Well, I'm afraid that it is and I'm very sorry and very angry because I wanted to tell you in person. Please forgive me.' And the result is that my mother and sister and I are much closer than we were ever before. And we were already very close.

ERIK (SWEDEN)

On the second day, I talked to my best friend about it. She was a woman, twenty years older than me, with two sons nearly my age. We met in nursing school and we had a really good friendship. I often stayed with them, because we studied together. I actually went into their family in a way.

I talked to her about it and she was sad at first. And then she said, 'Well, we just have to take some precautions, that's all – if you forget your shaving things at home, you don't borrow the boys' and so on.' And, just practical things, if I cut myself in the kitchen, she said just find out what we should do. She was a great help to me.

But there can also be very negative reactions.

ANGELA (SCOTLAND)

After I left the doctors, I went home to tell my husband. I went into the house, he was sitting at the fire. I said, 'I've got something to tell you, I've been told that I've got HIV.' He said, 'And how do they know? How did they find out? So you've got HIV and the doctors are just telling you now! And I've been sleeping with you all this time. I've been in gaol, so it's impossible that I've given it to you. You must have given it to me.' Well, he is non-tested so he doesn't even know.

There was no concern on his part really, he was just so angry. He put all the blame on me. He went on and on and said, 'You'd better get the doctors sued.' That was his concern, get the doctors sued. And then, 'You'd better not let anybody know.' He didn't want people to know that there was a chance that he had it, so I was to keep my mouth shut about myself. I wasn't to tell anybody and that was it.

I just felt really hurt. This man is supposed to love me and I don't know how he can love anybody, treating me like that, making me feel like a leper. He's supposed to be the closest person to me and he doesn't want that I tell anybody else. It was just so scary.

PARENTS

Some people have easy relationships with their parents, sharing their hopes and fears readily with them. But many find this relationship full of tensions. Telling parents of a life-threatening disease is clearly very difficult. First, there is the matter of finding the right time.

SARAH (ENGLAND)

My father had been asking me for a long time. He knows me really well and he'd be sat in the kitchen and he'd say, 'What's wrong? What's wrong, my love? What are you worrying about?' And I said, 'I'm fine, it's nothing.' I just wanted to tell them so much. I really wanted their love, their unconditional love. It doesn't matter the state of me or what I'd done or anything, that was what I wanted.

I'd told my brother. I've always been very close to him, so I told him first. He was really upset, he kept saying, 'I wish it was me, you haven't done anything to deserve this.' Then he couldn't face my parents because he knew this about me. Three weeks after I told him, I phoned him up after work and said, 'Tonight's the night.' And he said, 'Good, do it.'

We got home and my mother was in bed and my father – I always used to go in and chat with them – I went in and sat on the side of the bed. My dad said, 'What is it? What's wrong?' And I just couldn't say it, it was just so hard. My dad held my hand and he just said, 'Look, come on, nothing can be that bad.' So I sort of blurted it out: 'I'm HIV-positive.' And they just cried and held me and asked if the children had the virus.

It was very strange. My dad's got a really dry sense of humour and we were laughing, crying, then he put his arms around me and said, 'All I can say is, thank God you're not pregnant!' Because usually I go in and say, 'Dad, I'm pregnant again.' My mum just held on to me and said, 'I won't let you die, we're all going to fight this together.' She was really strong.

They were just wonderful. So supportive. They were cuddling me and holding me – when you're HIV you don't get touched – it was just so important. It was what I needed, to have somebody. I needed to talk and talk.

I always was close to all my family. The thing that has changed is that they're much more open about their problems. Whereas before, they wouldn't tell me things, they confide in me – to do with business and emotionally. So we're all much more open about everything.

And my brother's bought a bigger house, so that if anything happens to me there's a home for my two younger children. After he did it, he said, 'There's always those rooms for anybody.' I was really touched.

Some parents are very supportive.

DAVID (ENGLAND)

I think the most difficult thing was telling my mother. She lived with me at the time. I was terribly depressed, she'd been away for a bit and came home and – I don't know why – I just burst into tears. She said, 'What is it?' and I started to tell her and she said, 'You're trying to tell me you're HIV-positive, aren't you, dear?'

She's eighty-three years old, she's great. That's been marvellous. I realized that it's not just about HIV, it's about my relationship with my mother. And everything about me.

She's very proud of me. She talks about it all the time. She's learnt a lot too. She comes to all our meetings. She can't hear very well, but last week we had about sixty people there and she said, 'I just love to be in the midst of you all, because I've never felt such love.' That's great. I'm sure she must think in the quietness of her heart, 'What the hell's going on? My gay son.' She's got all that as well.

IMRAT (MALAYSIA)

I had very good support from my family. They said, 'You are part of the family, you are the son in the family, why should you be treated as a different person?' They make me think I am one of them, that I am still important in the family. And they make me feel that it's okay to have what I have, there's nothing wrong in it. It's just another disease that not many people know about.

I did feel very good that my family understands me, because if *they* didn't understand me, who else *could*? It makes me feel wanted, appreciated, even though I had the infection. To know that your family's not rejecting you, but they're supporting you in every way they can.

My family knew I was gay only when I told them I had HIV. They had to adjust to that. They did not talk about it, they did not ask me any questions about it. I told my mum and she said that it doesn't matter. She said, 'I always suspected that you were gay, because you always had calls from guys and letters from men and none from girls.' I had a very bad fight with my brother-in-law, who said he cannot accept that I'm gay, he wants to change me to straight. But it doesn't really matter, because my immediate family understands it.

TWENTY-FOUR

STAT

Najam Mughal

My work lies in between.
It skirts the main event.
It trails between cough and cure and appointments never kept.
It calibrates the basis,
That enumerates the waiting,
To enervate the point size of the jaded banner press.

My work is residue:
The fallout of the process between due date and death;
The confetti trace of health red tape;
The litter of care evidence.

These numbers I coalesce, code and quantify
I pattern the correlations
Between:
Health and wealth;
Births and deaths;
Change and time.

And the masticated statistics are fed back
To the battlefield of main events.

And the process begins again.

Source: Morley, D (ed.) *The Gift. New writing for the NHS*. Exeter: Stride Publications, 2002. Reproduced by permission.

PART III

THE PHYSICAL CONTEXT OF CARE

INTRODUCTION

Liz Forbat

The importance of bodies and the physical nature of encounters in health and social care seem obvious. Yet, how often do you hear about patients left in undignified positions, with only curtains to preserve their dignity, of social care staff forgetting to offer reassuring eye contact or a gentle touch, and doctors being physically threatened by patients? Embodiment and physicality are central and critical but all too often passed off as too ordinary for serious consideration. But because they permeate throughout encounters they require special attention. Experiences of pain, of soothing touch, of the senses, of movement, of beds and scratchy sheets, of heat and cold are all embodied, physical dimensions that impact upon the experience of health and social care. If their importance and meaning are lost in communicative encounters both practitioners and service users can pay high prices.

In this section a broad range of personal experiences and more academic musings are offered, which reflect widely and deeply on bodies. This includes the physicality of care exchanges, epitomised in ideas about how relationships are mediated through the physical nature of bodies and environments.

The range of accounts highlights the need to consider the importance of bodies, or, more broadly, physicality, in how care is delivered and received in health and social care settings. These embodied elements hold important possibilities for communication, spanning from childhood to older age. Some of this is in the 'obvious' way that much medical care is mediated through the body. People's bodies get sick, illness involves visible and invisible physical changes and care may involve touch. There are also other less obvious ways that physicality affects health and social care, for example the meaning and impact of the location of caregiving – whether in a person's own home, or a nursing home, or in their adult child's home. Bodies and the senses also enable people to play out different identities. Whether consciously or unconsciously, our bodies and physicality communicate all the time. They convey if a person is white or black, fat or thin, male or female, and act as cues to others about being strong, in control, nauseous, or scared.

The opening account from Linda Grant launches into a clearly embodied reflection on her mother and their relationship, as she describes the impact and onset of her mother's dementia. What is prioritised first in this account is how seeing her mother's body prompts her to reflect on her biography, marking out ideas of intimacy, domesticity, sexuality, loss and how social contexts such as dieting and grief impact on her body. It shows Grant's own emotional response to witnessing her mother's nakedness, and her mother's position as she tries on clothes in a shop changing-room. Then the account changes. The reader's gaze is no longer directed at the body. Grant points to the complex web of illnesses and relationships and how her mother's body and mind are experienced, as she reveals that her mother is troubled at a level of physicality, associated with her dementia.

Yasmin Gunaratnam's poem looks at the opportunities for tenderness and agony in paying close attention to bodies and the experience of care. As with Grant's piece, gender and sexuality become focal, but this time they are combined with strong images of 'race'. This powerful poem speaks the man's emotional responses to loss. His grief is both physical and relational: 'Do I miss her? He laughs': 'the glinting blade'. His communication is strongly evocative. However, this is offered up as a paradox, since the poet suggests that he is silent, but the reader catches a sharp, but fleeting glimpse of his story. This silence is not because there are not strong communicative messages; but because the signs he gives are not interpreted. Silence is the product of the others around him; it is they who render his experiences lost. This idea is represented in other extracts elsewhere in this book, for example by the patients in Ghada Karmi's account in Part I.

Sue Spurr's piece reflects on an encounter between her Aunty Jean and a doctor, and offers reflections on the importance of physicality to the business of getting on with life. The stark question posed in the title – 'Which would you prefer – a dislocated hip or wear a brace?' – is addressed through a critical appraisal of the doctor's communication with Aunty Jean. The tension between professional and service user is exemplified in how the treatment of a condition or illness becomes the primary marker of her life, rather than treatment enabling her to get on and live her life.

The need to consider wholeness in treating conditions continues as Tom Kitwood reflects on communication. Writing primarily about dementia he focuses on relationships, and how holism applies across different health and social care needs. In particular he highlights the importance of the psychological embodiment of the relationship and how power can be used to help or hinder communication. This connects with the poetry quoted in John Killick's contribution in Part II.

Lynne Murray and Liz Andrew's work offers lived examples of how infants embody communication. Their interactions are non-verbal and yet highly meaningful as gestures, facial movements and noises are interpreted and acted upon by other children, and especially by adults.

The ideas about subtle and non-verbal communication carry through to Jean-Dominique Bauby's piece, which offers two extreme examples of communication and interaction that are forcefully affected by his physical state of near total paralysis. His commentary suggests that finding ways of maintaining and enhancing communication was critical in how professionals related to him. Similar points are made by Oliver Sacks' account of receiving treatment for his broken leg in Part IV, where the link between care, physicality and relationships is made.

Cecil Helman's 'The radiological eye' continues the theme of enhancing communication in care settings, prompting thought about the impact of technology on the kind of communications that are now possible with and about bodies. It also illuminates a more complex way of viewing bodies, and in revealing messages behind the skin, it offers metaphors on the features shaping medical encounters. Niamh Merc's image continues this interest in technology, where care and embodiment are projected onto a figure depicting the ways in which people relate to bodies. Merc illustrates the polarities between a tactile sense of care and the estrangement created by mechanising care and relationships.

Two survivors of sexual abuse then offer very different perspectives on physicality. Death, distress and loneliness all have leading roles in these accounts, but through the act of communicating these deeply and painfully embodied reactions, come healing and comfort. For one author, dance becomes a way of being free, and for redefining her body and physicality not as something that has been abused, but a cathartic and expressive tool. As with infants, the non-verbal expression is packed solid with meaning. The second author, again describing trauma at a physical and emotional level, gives herself permission to describe and re-describe her experiences in different ways. In doing so she is liberated from the straitjacket of having only one version of her life to tell, one way of interpreting her relationship with her father and younger sister.

Marc Dugain's piece develops the theme of physicality in family and community relationships. The emotional pain of seeing himself through his family's eyes is followed by a trip into a village, facing strangers with the support of his friends. Marking the difference between private encounters with family and public ones with others, brings forth the importance of broad understandings of the physical environment and how this mediates and impacts upon communication. The ideas of space and physical locations are extended in Jennifer Hockey's poem. 'Care in the community' is a journey through the landscape of her father's life, the physical setting of Beverley, Yorkshire strongly evocative of a sense of belonging and a sense of the importance of home and comfort as her dad's death becomes evident.

Lastly there is an account of a woman who died shortly after writing about her 'deadly disease'. A desire to skip round the room jars against her anger at her body letting her down. But through the trauma of an intensely painful and debilitating condition, she finds solace in her good days, and the knowledge that her children have the promise of plans for their futures. These dreams leave behind her distressing experience of embodiment.

Each of these pieces offers a compelling contribution to the idea that there is vast potential in indicating the opportunities to communicate and liberate in positions of harm, fear and pain by attending to bodies, senses and physicality. They highlight the importance, for professionals and service users alike, in attending to the physical nature of care delivery and how this can be so easily compromised, and rectified, by attending to embodiment and physicality.

TWENTY-FIVE

'REMIND ME WHO I AM, AGAIN'
– EXTRACT 1

Linda Grant

In the changing room, she undresses. I remember the body I had seen in the bath when I was growing up, the convex belly from two Caesarean births that my sister used to think was like a washing-up bowl. The one that I have now, myself. She used to hold hers in under her clothes by that rubberized garment called a roll-on, a set of sturdy elasticized knickers. She had been six-and-a-half stone when she got married, which rose to ten stone after bearing her daughters, and she would spend twenty years adhering to the rules of Weight Watchers without ever noticeably losing a pound. Then she more or less stopped eating when my father died, apart from cakes and sweets and toast with low-calorie marge, on which regimen she shed two stone and twice was admitted to hospital suffering from dehydration.

As she removes her skirt, I turn my head away. It is enough to bear witness to the pornography of her left arm, a swollen sausage encased in a beige rubber bandage, the legacy of a pioneering mid-eighties operation for breast cancer which removed her lymph glands. The armpit is hollow.

The ensemble is in place when I look back. The pencil skirt, a size ten, is an exact fit but the blouse (also a ten) is a little too big, billowing round her hips, which is a shame for it is beautiful, in heavy matt silk with white over-stitching along the button closings.

And now my mother turns to me in rage, no longer placid and obedient, not the sweet little old age pensioner that shop assistants smile at seeing her delight in her new jacket.

Fury devours her. 'I *will* not wear this blouse, you will not *make* me wear this blouse.' She bangs her fist against the wall and (she is the only person I have ever seen do this) she stamps her foot, just like a character from one of

Source: Grant, L. *Remind Me Who I am, Again*. London: Granta Publications, 1998.
Reproduced by permission.

my childhood comics or a bad actress in an amateur production.

'What's the matter with it?'

She points to the collar. 'I'm not having anyone see me in this. It shows up my neck.'

I understand for the first time why, on this warm July day as well as every other, she is wearing a scarf knotted beneath her chin. I had thought her old bones were cold, but it is vanity. My mother was seventy-eight the previous week. 'Go and see if they've got it in a smaller size,' she orders.

My patient nephew is sitting beneath a mannequin outside watching the women come and go. There are very few eleven-year-old boys in the world who would spend a day of the school holidays traipsing around John Lewis with their aunt and their senile gran looking for clothes but let's face it, he has inherited the shopping gene. He's quite happy there, sizing up the grown ladies coming out the changing rooms to say to their friends, 'What do you think? Is it too dressy?' or 'I wonder what Ray's sister will be wearing. I'll kill her if it's cream.'

'Are you all right?' He gives me the thumbs-up sign. There is no size eight on the rack and I return empty-handed. My mother is standing in front of the mirror regarding herself: her fine grey hair, her hazel eyes, her obstinate chin, the illusory remains of girlish prettiness not ruined or faded or decayed but withered. Some people never seem to look like grown-ups but retain their childish faces all their lives and just resemble elderly infants. My mother did become an adult once but then she went back to being young again; young with lines and grey hair. Yet when I look at her I don't see any of it. She's just my mother, unchanging, the person who tells you what to do.

'Where've you been?' she asks, turning to me. 'This blouse is too big round the neck. Go and see if they've got it in a smaller size.'

'That's what I've been doing. They haven't.'

'Oh.'

So we continue to admire the skirt and the jacket and wait for the seamstress to arrive, shut up together in our little cubicle where once, long ago, my mother would say to me: 'You're not having it and that's final. I wouldn't be seen dead with you wearing something like that. I don't care if it's all the rage. I don't care if everyone else has got one. You can't.'

My mother fingers the collar on the blouse. 'I'm not wearing this, you know. They can't make me wear it. I'm not going to the wedding if I've got to wear this blouse.'

'Nobody's going to make you wear it. We'll look for something else.'

'I've got an idea. Why don't you see if they have it in a smaller size?'

'I've looked already. There isn't one. This is the last . . .'

'No, I must interrupt you. I've just thought, do you think they've got it in a smaller size?'

'That's what I'm trying to tell you. They haven't got one.'

Her shoulders sag in disappointment.

TWENTY-SIX

THE BED

Yasmin Gunaratnam

Intent concern accompanied the glinting blade
That sliced from hip to hip.
A tributary
Meandering down into dry recesses of manliness.
A cut so deep, so low
Folds of distinction reopen.
Hard layers. Moist untouched spaces.
Shiny black skin. Striated muscle.
Prowess.
Flow into tired, needy sinews of a pure new
Softness.

He has a story to tell.
He doesn't know
How.
Since she gone, he says
He has not slept one night in that bed.
Do I miss her?
He laughs.
Perhaps. But I have to break my mind to the condition, in'it?
And the reason, most of my reason is because
Through my tablets, I pass water often.
To walk from the bed is a longer
Movement.
On this chair
Out here
I just roll off, pee in the bucket.
It's easier.

And that bed is wide. Very wide.
At night.

In the shadows of nightfall
He feels the knife.
This time in his heart.
Quivering. Shimmering.
In this place of dislocation
Contorted emasculation
He marks his loss. Silently,
With truth.
Rolling the saltiness around his mouth.

He leans forward slowly
Pisses into the bucket.

Relieved.

TWENTY-SEVEN

AUNTY JEAN

Sue Spurr

Which would you prefer – a dislocated hip or wear a brace?

As I climbed the two steps up to her two bed roomed bungalow I wondered if there is another 83-year-old woman like my Aunty Jean? I'm greeted by the smell of mothballs and a fascinating assortment of her life. Aware that I'm entering a different world I try to adapt. The effect of things everywhere carefully packaged and covered is claustrophobic and the grandfather clock seems to chime a message of 'don't touch'. Yet it feels neat and clean as opposed to the chaos and cobwebs of my family home. The cupboards are filled with dried food and tins – sufficient to keep my family of five going for years – belying a siege mentality and a throwback to her life in Labarador as nurse with the Grenfell Mission.

Having no partner she turns her life to suit herself but I wouldn't call her selfish. She's this strange mix of timidity and ineffective assertion which is often typical of women of her generation and middle class background. She doesn't grumble much about all her ailments which she bears with increasing difficulty as the years pass. Her eyesight is failing fast (some sort of degenerative eye condition beginning 'M' – macula or something); she's been plagued by depression all her life and recently she's had to cope with an unsuccessful – in that it has dislocated twice through no real fault of hers it seems – hip joint replacement.

Thirty years ago Jean would climb the mountains that surround her Lake District home with the ease of a mountain goat. Physically she was robust and strong. In this respect she is now the very antithesis of her former self. She is shrunken, her head tilts so far forward it touches her chest and she can just about put one leg in front of the other. Much of Jean's day is spent shuffling from one room to another sorting out her possessions and wondering if she'll see anyone. The phone is her only connection with the outside world for most of the day until her carer comes at

7pm-ish to help her prepare for the long night ahead. There are two steps up to her house – how much longer can she mount these steps?

After her hip dislocated the first time (she passed out and fell) she was fitted with a contraption – a brace – designed to keep the hip joint from dislocating. It does the job perfectly that is if you don't mind not sleeping, any movement restricted to a kind of shuffle, not being able to get on a bus, not being able to have a bath – in effect being reduced to such a humiliating state that there are times when life really doesn't seem worth living.

It was about 9am one October morning when Jean and I set off to the hospital to meet the orthopaedic consultant surgeon – Mr R. We'd planned what we were going to say and our plan was to initiate a discussion that although the brace is protecting Jean's hip it is also causing problems.

But when we got into his consulting room, it was clear from the start that Mr R. does all the talking leaving very little room for questions; keeps very focussed on what he thinks is important and moves people on and out as if they are on a conveyor belt. I also realised when Mr R. said, 'Well I know about your hip but what about your knee?' that I'd not grasped one fairly important fact – that this visit was actually about Jean's knee and not about her hip. Within seconds he'd ordered her to walk up and down and she shuffled obediently the length of the room. A few more seconds and he pronounced her knee to be very swollen. Hmm. After much manipulating and talking over her gasps of pain Mr R. confidently diagnosed that it is probably arthritis. He offered Jean an 'injection to make it more comfortable' there and then and without waiting for a reply set off to get his needle. I hissed at Jean 'Is this what you want?' I felt the full brunt of Mr R's glare. Somehow Jean managed to ask what was in the injection. After ascertaining that the injection involved cortisone, Jean said 'No' as she'd never had cortisone and wasn't sure that she was about to start. Mr R. shrugged and said that she'd have to put up with the pain then. He then suggested that Jean be put on a list for 'hoovering out the knee' which would mean a short stay in hospital. She agreed to this and is now waiting four or five months for this.

I wanted to say 'Her knee is obviously very sore. I do wonder if it's made worse by the brace (which is supporting the hip joint on the opposite side)' but my courage failed me. Somehow this man required people to do as you were told and ask no questions. I stood limply by wondering what was going to happen next.

It was clear that as far as Mr R. was now concerned the consultation was over and he began summing up. We'd had our ten minute slot. I could see the conveyor belt moving.

Suddenly Jean assumed her ineffective assertive mode and I heard her saying 'I guess I have to keep this brace on till next Easter?' to which Mr R. replied 'Which would you prefer – a dislocated hip or a brace?'

I could feel my hackles rising.

Jean's reply was a resounding 'A dislocated hip' and I don't think she was joking.

Mr R. failed completely to hear the significance of Jean's response. I think he saw her as being facetious and proceeded to give a lecture on the dangers of dislocated hips and the sense of wearing the brace. All very true, of course, but isn't the dilemma clear – if the brace is left on, then the hip is relatively safe but Jean's emotional and physical wellbeing plummets; on the other hand, whereas if the brace is taken off completely then despite an increased risk at least she would hopefully feel a bit better.

I took a deep breath and I decided to try and get him to see the situation more widely and asked him if this sort of treatment was the most appropriate given that it is giving Jean a great deal of discomfort particularly at night and how wearing the brace is actually wearing her down both emotionally and physically. My words tumbled out fast and incoherently. I could feel my left leg shaking and I had serious thoughts that if my heart beat any faster I might need to be directed to cardiology for a check up on the way out. He certainly didn't want to be challenged and I got the 'benefit' of another one of his little lectures on dislocated hips. I heard Jean trying to tell him about how it had become dislocated but he wasn't in 'receiver mode' it seemed.

I could sense that Jean was subdued. Mr R. was backing out of the room.

However, all of a sudden he said 'OK go home and take off the brace'. It was all or nothing with this man. I think we both felt quite unsettled as he didn't seem to want to discuss any option other than what is prescribed. We were dismissed and emerged from his consulting room a bit dazed and unclear about what to do next.

I felt extremely frustrated that we had wanted to ask all sorts of questions but the 'opportunity' was gone. I wasn't happy or convinced that it was sensible for it to come off altogether. Perhaps it would be better for it to come off at night and on during the day to allow her to gradually regain her confidence? Although no doubt Mr R. would be writing to the GP I couldn't be confident that he was interested in helping out with the practicalities of how Jean was going to manage getting the brace on and off. Carers are not trained to take braces on or off and therefore might not be willing to do it. I could see a problem looming.

We had fish and chips after leaving the hospital. Jean seemed confused and out of sorts. The whole thing had been an exhausting and disabling experience. Was it that difficult to enable someone to take part in their own decision making when it had a direct and significant bearing on their life?

I persuaded Jean that we must call in at her GP practice on the way home and see if we could sort out some sort of support for her.

At the surgery I met Sister Brown the district nurse. She said, being a sensible person, she could see both sides – that of Mr R. but she could also see the effect of wearing the brace was having on Jean. She didn't feel confident about taking the brace on and off herself but she promised that she would arrange a joint meeting between herself, someone from the hospital and Jean and the carer and try and get something organised. Everyone agreed that the answer is not to remove the brace completely but try it off at night and on during the day for a while.

The receptionist at the surgery told me that the CPN had been trying to get in touch with Jean all day – apparently she had had an appointment at 1pm. In fact when I mentioned this to Jean she said that she hadn't forgotten and had left a message to say that she wouldn't be in – unfortunately the message never got through. I asked Jean if I should ring and make another appointment and explain where we'd been and she let me do this. The CPN has my number as a contact number if need be. I explained everything to the CPN so she is in the know and afterwards wondered if I should book an appointment for me too . . .

Finally I headed down the M6 at about 5pm after a cup of tea contemplating what Mr R. would say if I'd had the courage to ask him 'Which would you prefer – a dislocated hip or wear a brace?'

TWENTY-EIGHT

THE EXPERIENCE OF DEMENTIA: IMPROVING CARE

Tom Kitwood

Although what follows is highly speculative, it is derived from careful observation; and . . . I am deliberately drawing on my own poetic fantasy. This imaginative account depicts the experience of a woman in her 80s who has severe cognitive impairments, and who is now in residential care.

You are in a garden, at the start of a summer's day. The air is warm and gentle, carrying the sweet scent of flowers, and a slight mist is floating around. You can't make out the shape of everything, but you are aware of some beautiful colours, blue, orange, pink and purple; the grass is green as emerald. You don't know where you are, but this doesn't matter. You somehow feel 'at home', and there is a sense of harmony and peace.

As you walk around, you become aware of other people. Several of them seem to know you; it is a joy to be greeted so warmly, and by name. There are one or two of them whom you feel sure you know well. And then there is that one special person. She seems so warm, so kind, so understanding. She must be your mother; how good it is to be back with her again. The flame of life now burns brightly and cheerfully within you. It hasn't always been like this. Somewhere, deep inside, there are dim memories of times of crushing loneliness and ice-cold fear. When that was, you do not know; perhaps it was in another life. Now there is company whenever you want it, and quietness when that is what you prefer. This is the place where you belong, with these wonderful people; they are like a kind of family.

The work that you do here is the best you have ever had. The hours are flexible, and the job is pleasant; being with people is what you have always

Source: Kitwood, T. *Dementia Reconsidered. The person comes first.* Buckingham: Open University Press, 1997. Reproduced by permission.

enjoyed. You can do the work at exactly your own pace, without any rush or pressure, and you can rest whenever you need. For instance there is that kind man who often comes to see you – by a strange coincidence his name is the same as that of your husband. He seems to need you, and to enjoy being with you. You, for your part, are glad to give time to being with him, his presence, strangely, gives you comfort.

As you pass by a mirror you catch a glimpse of a person who looks quite old. Is it your grandmother, or that person who used to live next door? Anyway, it is good to see her too. Then you begin to feel tired; you find a chair and you sit down, alone. Soon you become aware of a chill around your heart, a sinking feeling in your stomach – the deadly fear is coming over you again. You are about to cry out, but then you see that kind mother-person, already there, sitting beside you. Her hand is held out towards you, waiting for you to grasp it. As you talk together, the fear evaporates like the morning mist, and you are again in the garden, relaxing in the golden warmth of the sun. You know it isn't heaven itself, but sometimes it feels as if it might be halfway there.

It is impossible to say, as yet, how many people might have this kind of experience if there were a serious and sustained attempt to meet their psychological needs. The project hasn't yet been tried on a large enough scale. Even at this time, however, we can be certain that many people will be more at ease with their limitations, more able to live without a historical sense of time or a geographical sense of place. They will feel far better supported, far less alone, in whatever suffering is unavoidable. They will have a new chapter in life, with its own special delights and pleasures. And finally, they will be more able to accept with tranquillity the coming of death.

[. . .]

Human existence, unfortunately, is far from idyllic. History reveals a continuing succession of organized acts of violence, cruelty, oppression and exploitation. Very few societies have found lasting ways of minimizing these abuses; the problems are particularly great where there is a gross imbalance of wealth and power. We have to face the fact that those finely developed capacities that human beings have for cooperation can be harnessed in highly destructive ways.

Much more prevalent and insidious, however, at least in 'civilized' society, are those subtle ways of demeaning and discounting the person that are incorporated into ordinary interaction: tiny remarks tinged with mockery or cruelty; exercises of social power; subtle manipulations; insinuations that the other is inadequate; avoidances of direct emotional contact. These often pass unnoticed at a conscious level, and are simply taken as 'normality'. A central part of the problem here is that very few people are able to give 'free attention' to one another for more than a few fleeting moments. New recruits to counselling courses often learn, with surprise and shock, how incompetent they are in active listening, and out of the whole population, these are the very people in whom this skill is likely to be relatively well developed.

The scene is a beach, on a day in the height of summer. In the background there are sounds of play and laughter, but a little girl aged 3 or 4 is crying piteously. Her parents are sitting nearby in their deckchairs. 'Stop that crying, or I'll give you something to cry for.' The child continues to wail. She is slapped on the leg. She cries some more, then slowly stifles her sobs. She moves a little further away from her parents, and begins to dig in the sand, alone.

This tiny episode is paradigmatic. In many people's eyes it would be construed as part of ordinary parenting. At a level below consciousness, perhaps the child learned some important lessons: that her innocent desire to play with others will be frustrated, that she must submit to parental power, that she would do well to conceal her feelings of anger and dismay. Through acts such as this her exquisite sensitivities are cauterized; her personality becomes imbued with wariness and psychological defence.

Observations along these lines have been made by many psychologists involved in some way with counselling and psychotherapy, for example Rogers (1961), Miller (1987) and Bradshaw (1990). In Buber's terms (1937), the problem is the repeated failure to meet a person as Thou, and the imposition of an I–It mode of relating. We have come to accept the diminution of persons as a norm in everyday life, and many people live in an interactional prison without ever recognizing the fact. The malignant social psychology which comes into the open so obviously in contexts such as dementia care is but an exaggerated and shameless form of the 'normal' social psychology of everyday life, whose malignant effect might be compared to that of low-level background radiation.

POSITIVE PERSON WORK

If we make a close observation of really good dementia care . . . it becomes clear that several different types of interaction are involved. Each one enhances personhood in a different way: strengthening a positive feeling, nurturing an ability, or helping to heal some psychic wound. The quality of interaction is warmer, more rich in feeling, than that of (British) everyday life. An episode that can be described in an ordinary way (reminiscing, going for a walk, having a meal, etc.) usually consists of a sequence of short-lived interactions of different types, like beads on a string. Sometimes the succession of interactions does not make up a social act of a recognizable kind; here it is as if the 'definition of the situation' changed on the way, and perhaps changed several times. Something very similar often happens in children's play.

The [10] different types of positive interaction that are outlined here form only a very provisional list. It is consistent with the ideas of workers who have developed and used the Quality of Interaction Schedule (Clarke and Bowling 1990; Dean *et al.* 1993). However, building on the observational method of Dementia Care Mapping, it provides a considerably higher level of detail. A full elaboration still awaits detailed research.

1 *Recognition* – Here a man or woman who has dementia is being acknowledged as a person, known by name, affirmed in his or her own uniqueness. Recognition may be achieved in a simple act of greeting, or in careful listening over a longer period – perhaps as a person describes an earlier part of his or her life. Recognition, though, is never purely verbal, and it need not involve words at all. One of the profoundest acts of recognition is simply the direct contact of the eyes.

2 *Negotiation* – The characteristic feature of this type of interaction is that people who have dementia are being consulted about their preferences, desires and needs, rather than being conformed to others' assumptions. Much negotiation takes place over simple everyday issues, such as whether a person feels ready to get up, or have a meal, or go outdoors. Skilled negotiation takes into account the anxieties and insecurities that often pervade the lives of people with dementia, and the slower rate at which they handle information. Negotiation gives even highly dependent people some degree of control over the care that they receive, and puts power back into their hands.

3 *Collaboration* – Here we gain a glimpse of two or more people aligned on a shared task, with a definite aim in view. The true meaning of collaboration is 'working together', and this may literally be the case; as, for example, in doing the same household chores. Less obviously, it can occur in contexts of personal care such as getting dressed, having a bath or going to the toilet. The hallmark of collaboration is that care is not something that is 'done to' a person who is cast into a passive role; it is a process in which their own initiative and abilities are involved.

4 *Play* – Whereas work is directed towards a goal, play in its purest form has no goal that lies outside the activity itself. It is simply an exercise in spontaneity and self-expression, an experience that has value in itself. Because of the sheer pressures of survival, and the disciplines of work, many adults have only poorly developed abilities in this area. A good care environment is one which allows these abilities to grow.

5 *Timalation* – This term refers to forms of interaction in which the prime modality is sensuous or sensual, without the intervention of concepts and intellectual understanding; for example through aromatherapy and massage. The word itself is a neologism, derived from the Greek word *timao* (I honour, and hence I do not violate personal or moral boundaries) and stimulation (with its connotations of sensory arousal). The significance of this kind of interaction is that it can provide contact, reassurance and pleasure, while making very few demands. It is thus particularly valuable when cognitive impairment is severe.

6   *Celebration* – The ambience here is expansive and convivial. It is not
    simply a matter of special occasions, but of any moment at which life is
    experienced as intrinsically joyful. Many people who have dementia,
    despite their suffering, retain the capacity to celebrate; perhaps it is
    even enhanced as the burdens of responsibility disappear. Celebration
    is the form of interaction in which the division between caregiver and
    cared-for comes nearest to vanishing completely; all are taken up into a
    similar mood. The ordinary boundaries of ego have become diffuse,
    and selfhood has expanded. In some mystical traditions, this is the
    meaning of spirituality.
7   *Relaxation* – Of all the forms of interaction, this is the one that has the
    lowest level of intensity, and probably also the slowest pace. It is pos-
    sible, of course, to relax in solitude, but many people with dementia,
    with their particularly strong social needs, are only able to relax when
    others are near them, or in actual bodily contact.

While each of the seven types of interaction that we have examined has a
strongly positive content, three others are more distinctly psychotherapeutic.

8   *Validation* – This term has a long history in psychotherapeutic work,
    going back some time before Naomi Feil made it famous in dementia
    care (e.g. Laing 1967). The literal meaning is to make strong or robust;
    to validate the experience of another is to accept the reality and power
    of that experience, and hence its 'subjective truth'. The heart of the
    matter is acknowledging the reality of a person's emotions and feelings,
    and giving a response on the feeling level. Validation involves a high
    degree of empathy, attempting to understand a person's entire frame of
    reference, even if it is chaotic or paranoid, or filled with hallucinations.
    When our experience is validated we feel more alive, more connected,
    and more real; there is every ground for supposing that this is true in
    dementia as well.
9   *Holding* – This, of course, is a metaphor, derived from the physical
    holding of a child who is in distress. To hold, in a psychological sense,
    means to provide a safe psychological space, a 'container'; here hidden
    trauma and conflict can be brought out; areas of extreme vulnerability
    exposed. When the holding is secure a person can know, in experience,
    that devastating emotions such as abject terror or overwhelming grief
    will pass, and not cause the psyche to disintegrate. Even violent anger
    or destructive rage, directed for a while at the person who is doing the
    holding, will not drive that person away. As in the case of childcare,
    psychological holding in any context may involve physical holding too.
10 *Facilitation* – At its simplest this means enabling a person to do what
    otherwise he or she would not be able to do, by providing those parts
    of the action – and only those – that are missing. Facilitation of this

kind merges into what I have called collaboration. The more truly psychotherapeutic interaction occurs when a person's sense of agency has been seriously depleted, or when action schemata have largely fallen apart. Perhaps all that is left is a hesitant move towards an action, or an elementary gesture. The task of facilitation now is to enable interaction to get started, to amplify it and to help the person gradually to fill it out with meaning. When this is done well there is a great sensitivity to the possible meanings in a person's movements, and interaction proceeds at a speed that is slow enough to allow meaning to develop.

Each of the types of interaction we have considered thus far represents a form of 'care', in the sense that the person with dementia is primarily at the receiving end, or is being actively drawn into the social world. There are some interactions, however, in which the situation is reversed; the person with dementia takes the leading role, and the caregiver is offering an empathic response. As with the other types of interaction, these might continue for several minutes, or be short-lived.
[. . .]

Good dementia care, then, has a kind of ecology, in which a variety of types of interaction merge into one another, and there is a continuing succession. We might imagine a natural forest of conifers, interspersed with patches of alpine meadow in which a hundred species are to be found in a few square yards. Poor care, in contrast, is dead and regimented; there are long periods of neglect, and small episodes of malignant social psychology fill a few of the spaces. We might think of a conifer plantation cultivated purely for the purposes of agribusiness, where the trees are in rows and almost nothing grows between them; there is virtually no sign of the grace and beauty of a natural system, and the atmosphere is dark and depressing.

REFERENCES

Bradshaw, J. (1990) *Homecoming*, London, Piatkus.

Buber, M. (1937) *I and Thou* (trans. by R. Gregor Smith), Edinburgh, Clark.

Clarke, P. and Bowling, A. (1990) 'Quality of everyday life in long-stay institutions for the elderly', *Social Science and Medicine*, Vol. 30, pp. 1201–10.

Dean, R., Proudfoot, R. and Lindesay, J. (1993) 'The Quality of Interaction Schedule (QUIS): development, reliability and use in the evaluation of two domus units', *International Journal of Geriatric Psychiatry*, Vol. 8, pp. 819–26.

Laing, R. D. (1967) *The Politics of Experience*, Harmondsworth, Penguin.

Miller, A. (1987) *The Drama of Being a Child*, London, Virago.

Rogers, C. R. (1961) *On Becoming a Person*, Boston, MA, Houghton Mifflin.

TWENTY-NINE

EXTRACT FROM 'THE SOCIAL BABY'

Lynne Murray and Liz Andrew

COMMUNICATION WITH PEOPLE

'Let's chat'

Babies are attracted to other people from birth and they quickly prefer the people who have become familiar. But the baby doesn't simply want to be near her family and their friends – she wants to share her experience with other people and interact with them!

Over the first few weeks the baby gradually becomes more active in her social contacts. She can be helped to enjoy 'chatting' with her social partners. In the first three months, the best distance for the baby to see someone's face in focus is 22 cm (9 in.), and it helps in the early weeks if the baby's head is well supported. Some babies find it more difficult than others to hold their head up, and they will need support for some time. This is particularly likely with babies who were born prematurely. Being aware of the baby's state is also important: if the baby is sleepy, hungry, or in pain, the last thing she will feel like is being sociable. If however, the baby is contented and alert, and in a comfortable position, she is likely to be keen to interact.

In the first weeks, the baby's active involvement in face-to-face communication is often rather fleeting, so, although she is very interested in other people, having prolonged 'conversations' is unusual. As the weeks go by, however, the baby will be able to remain interested for longer periods; eye-

Source: Murray L, Andrews, L. *The Social Baby*. Richmond: The Children's Project, 2000, pp. 46–51. Reproduced by permission. www.childrenproject.co.uk

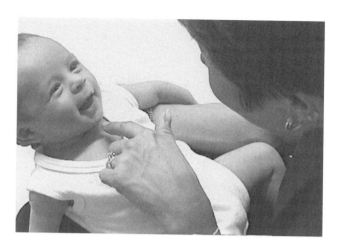

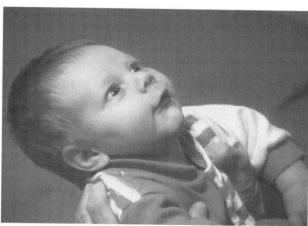

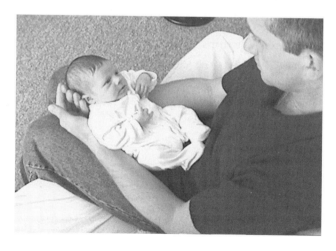

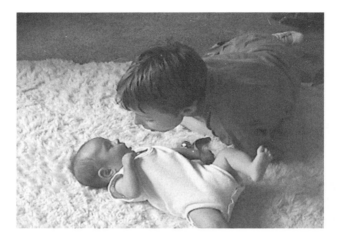

to-eye contact can be sustained, smiling becomes more reliable, and the baby can begin to play a more active role in interactions.

On such occasions the baby's mouth is often very mobile, with her tongue coming forward out of her mouth, or pushing into her lower lip, or she may open her mouth wide. These bursts of active effort can last for a number of seconds. It seems as though the baby is trying to talk and, indeed, some scientists have called this behaviour 'pre-speech' because, although not often accompanied by sound in the first weeks, it seems to serve the role of speech, reflecting the baby's efforts to communicate. Even the baby's limb movements can form a part of the baby's social behaviour, her arms rising, and her fingers often opening and pointing in concert when her mouthing reaches its peak. At such times, parents often make remarks such as 'That's a good story you're telling me', sensing that the baby's behaviour reflects her impulse to be sociable. When the partner picks up on the baby's cues and responds, this sustains the baby's involvement, and prolonged, two-way 'conversations' can take place in which the baby and her partner take turns watching being active in the dialogue.

The baby's active communication 1

Natasha, 3 weeks

Natasha is only three weeks old, and her use of facial expression, mouthing and tongue movements for communication is still rather limited. Nevertheless, she watches her mother's face with fascination, and her interest and enthusiasm are also apparent in her hand and arm movements, as she reaches and gestures towards her mother.

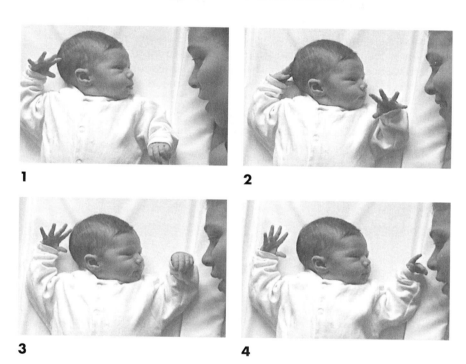

The baby's active communication 2

Zak, 5 weeks

When alert and content, with head well supported, babies of just a few weeks old often appear keen to participate in what look like 'conversations' with a sympathetic partner. The baby communicates with a rich range of facial expressions, tongue movements and active shapings of the mouth that are often accompanied by hand and arm gestures. This kind of activity, although not often vocal in the first weeks, has been termed 'pre-speech',* since it seems to serve the same function as speech in adult conversation – and indeed, parents will often make comments such as 'You've got a lot to tell me today', that support this interpretation.

Here we see Zak totally absorbed in communication with Liz. Initially, he watches her intently, but quickly begins to take an active role. He shapes his mouth in different positions, and his tongue is very mobile, moving inside his mouth, but also protruding beyond his lips. At times, as he raises his arms, he will extend his index finger at the peak of the arm movement, as if making a particularly important point! Long before words emerge, essential elements of human engagement are in place.

*The term 'pre-speech' was coined by Colwyn Trevarthen.

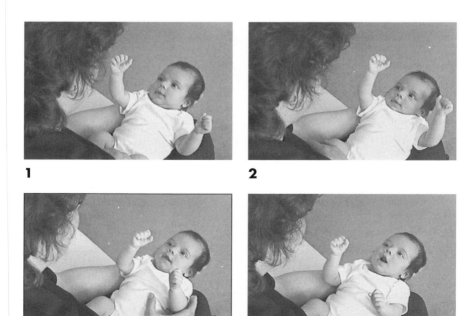

1

2

3

4

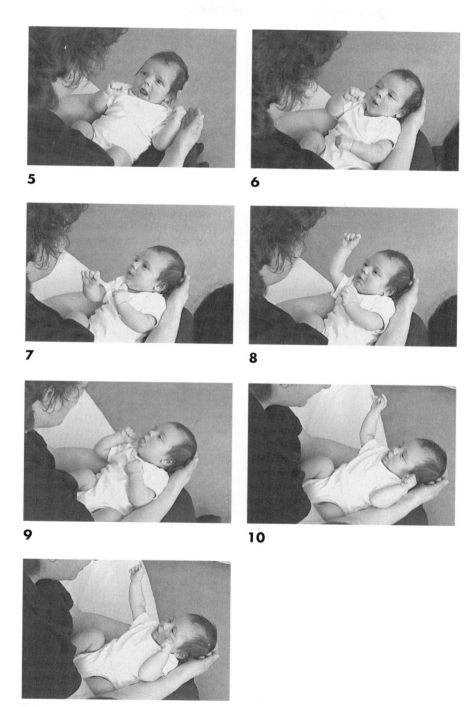

5

6

7

8

9

10

11

THIRTY

EXTRACT FROM 'THE DIVING-BELL AND THE BUTTERFLY'

Jean-Dominique Bauby

GUARDIAN ANGEL

The identity badge pinned to Sandrine's white tunic says 'Speech Therapist', but it should read 'Guardian Angel'. She is the one who set up the communication code without which I would be cut off from the world. But alas! While most of my friends have adopted the system, here at the hospital only Sandrine and one lady psychologist use it. So I usually have the skimpiest arsenal of facial expressions, winks and nods to ask people to shut the door, turn on a tap, lower the volume on the TV, or fluff up a pillow. I do not succeed every time. As the weeks go by, this forced solitude has allowed me to acquire a certain stoicism and to realize that the hospital staff are of two kinds: the majority, who would not dream of leaving the room without first attempting to decipher my SOS messages; and the less conscientious minority, who make their getaway pretending not to notice my distress signals. Like that heartless oaf who switched off the Bordeaux–Munich football game at half-time, saying 'Goodnight!' with a finality that left no hope of appeal. Quite apart from the practical drawbacks, this inability to communicate is somewhat wearing. Which explains the gratification I feel twice daily when Sandrine knocks, pokes her small chipmunk face through the door and at once sends all gloomy thoughts packing. The invisible and eternally imprisoning cocoon seems less oppressive.

Speech therapy is an art that deserves to be more widely known. You

Source: Bauby, J-D. *The Diving Bell and the Butterfly*. London: Forth Estate Ltd, 1997.
Reproduced by permission.

cannot imagine the acrobatics your tongue mechanically performs in order to produce all the sounds of a language. Just now I am struggling with the letter 'l', a pitiful admission for an editor-in-chief who cannot even pronounce the name of his own magazine! On good days, between coughing fits, I muster enough energy and wind to be able to puff out one or two phonemes. On my birthday Sandrine managed to get me to pronounce the whole alphabet more or less intelligibly. I could not have had a better present. I heard those twenty-six letters wrenched from the void by a hoarse voice emanating from the mists of time. The exhausting exercise left me feeling like a caveman discovering language for the first time. Sometimes the phone interrupts our work, and I take advantage of Sandrine's presence to be in touch with loved ones, to intercept and catch passing fragments of life, the way you catch a butterfly. My daughter Céleste tells me of her adventures with her pony. In five months she will be nine. My father tells me how hard it is to stay on his feet. He is fighting undaunted through his ninety-third year. These two are the outer links of the chain of love which surrounds and protects me. I often wonder about the effect of these one-way conversations on those at the other end of the line. I am overwhelmed by them. How dearly I would love to be able to respond with something other than silence to these tender calls. I know that some of them find it unbearable. Sweet Florence refuses to speak to me unless I first breathe noisily into the receiver which Sandrine holds glued to my ear. 'Are you there, Jean-Do?' she asks anxiously over the air.

And I have to admit that at times I do not know any more.

VOICE OFF

I have known gentler awakenings. When I came to that late-January morning the hospital ophthalmologist was leaning over me and sewing my right eyelid shut with a needle and thread, just as if he were darning a sock. Irrational terror swept over me. What if this man got carried away and sewed up my left eye as well, my only link to the outside world, the only window to my cell, the one tiny opening of my cocoon? Luckily, as it turned out, I wasn't plunged into darkness. He carefully packed his sewing kit away in padded tin boxes. Then, in the tones of a prosecutor demanding a maximum sentence for a repeat offender, he barked out: 'Six months!' I fired off a series of questioning signals with my working eye, but this man – who spent his days looking into other people's pupils – was apparently unable to interpret a simple look. He was the very model of the couldn't-care-less doctor, arrogant, brusque, sarcastic, the kind who summons his patients for 8.00 a.m., arrives at 9.00, and departs at 9.05 after giving each one forty-five seconds of his precious time. Physically he looked like Dennis the Menace, with a big round head, short body and a fidgety manner. Already disinclined to chat with normal patients, he turned thoroughly evasive in dealing with ghosts of my ilk, apparently incapable of finding words to offer the slightest explanation. But I finally discovered why he had put a six-month seal on my eye: the lid was no longer fulfilling its function as a protective cover, and I ran the risk of an ulcerated cornea.

As the weeks went by I wondered whether the hospital employed such an ungracious character deliberately – to serve as a focal point for the veiled mistrust the medical profession always arouses in long-term patients. A kind of scapegoat in other words. If he leaves Berck, which seems likely, who will be left for me to sneer at? I shall no longer have the solitary and innocent pleasure of hearing his eternal question, 'Do you see double?' and of replying – deep inside – 'Yes, I see two assholes, not one.'

I need to feel strongly, to love and to admire, just as desperately as I need to breathe. A letter from a friend, a Balthus painting on a postcard, or a page of Saint-Simon give meaning to the passing hours. But to keep my mind sharp, to avoid slumping into resigned indifference, I maintain a level of resentment and anger, neither too much nor too little, just as a pressure-cooker has a safety-valve to keep it from exploding.

And while we're on the subject, *The Pressure-Cooker* could be a title for the play I may write one day, based on my experiences here. I've also thought of calling it *The Eye*, and of course *The Cocoon*. You already know the plot and the setting. A hospital room in which Mr L, a family man in the prime of life, is learning to live with locked-in syndrome brought on by a serious cerebro-vascular accident. The play follows Mr L's adventures in the medical world and his shifting relationship with his wife, his children, his friends, and his associates from the leading advertising agency he helped to found. Ambitious, somewhat cynical, heretofore a stranger to failure, Mr L takes his first steps into distress, sees all the certainties that buttressed him collapse, and discovers that his nearest and dearest are strangers. We could carry this slow transformation as far as the front seats of the balcony, where a voice off would reproduce Mr L's unspoken inner monologue as he faces each new situation. All that is left is to write the play. I have the final scene already. The stage is in darkness, except for a halo of light around the bed in centre-stage. Night-time. Everyone sleeps. Suddenly Mr L, inert since the curtain first rose, throws aside sheets and blankets, jumps from the bed and walks around the eerily lit stage. Then it grows dark again and you hear the voice off – Mr L's inner voice – one last time:

'Shit! It was only a dream!'

THIRTY-ONE

THE RADIOLOGICAL EYE

Cecil Helman

There are four luminescent panels in the room, in a silver frame on the table, and rows of black books on a shelf, and journals, and crushed Styrofoam cups with the barnacles of yesterday's coffee. Rectangles of X-Ray film are pinned to the panels, a dark parade of skulls and skeletons in the underwater light of the little room, in the white-tiled building with many corridors. This is the radiology room, the room of white bones and empty flesh.

It is almost a century now since Wilhelm Conrad Röntgen discovered the invisible X-Ray, and at the end of 1895 published his monograph – *Eine neue Art von Strahlen* ('On a New Kind of Rays') – in the German city of Würzburg. A few days earlier, on the 22nd December, in a moment of medical history, he had passed these new kind of rays right through his wife's opened hand, and then onto a photographic plate.

We can still see the ghostly outlines of Frau Röntgen's hand, with the dark finger bones and the large oval ring, and still they throw their long shadows over our perceptions of the human body. For the first time the eye travels to within the living body, and peers around inside, without ever tearing open its envelope of skin. The body is transparent now, and because of that some part of the mind, too, loses its solidity and becomes more permeable to the outside eye.

The aim of radiology is still the uncovering of secrets, the revelation of mysteries that are masked by flesh. With the aid of radiology you can 'see through' or into someone, but their selfhood is dissolved by your gaze. Look at the screen now, and there is no one there. All that remains of the individual are the imperfections of form: a broken bone, a swollen heart, a twisted womb, a back hunched over like a question mark. The human

Source: Helman, C. *Body Myths*. London: Chatto & Windus, 1991.
Reproduced by permission.

beings have all disappeared, shrunk to the banal cartoons of Hallowe'en. Stare at these too long and even they will vanish, as the bones weaken, and the cells of the marrow become malevolent and multiply.

But now look a little closer at the screen, for seen through the radiological eye your body can encode all the cycles and seasons of the year. Within the human frame the rays reveal a natural landscape of light and shadow, a chiaroscuro of suffering or health. It is a paradoxical world, a world turned inside-out and upside-down. The topographies of skin and expression have gone, so have all the solidities of organs, and muscles and tendons. Only their spectral, translucent shadows remain on the screen, still outlined in skin.

In these shadows we can recognize the echoes of midnight or noon, autumn or spring. There is the clear summer light of a healthy limb or lung, or the little white flakes of infection scattered over a dark chest, like a snowfall at the beginning of a winter's night.

There is the 'rib cage', as it is called, with its most famous inmates: the pulsing boot-shaped heart, the long conduit of the oesophagus, the spongy irregular lungs, and the large blood vessels arching backwards to behind the heart. In radiology, as in language, here in the cage is the heart of the matter, the seat of metaphor. Here is the universal flesh-box of the emotions, and within it – whether hard, soft, warm or cold, broken or black – vibrates that little personality, hidden within the Self.

In this *mundus inversus* of hidden forms, the hollows of the body tell their own story. It is a text of spaces and absences, of empty shapes that are filled with meaning, like the plaster casts of vanished corpses in the hard larva of Pompeii, or the shadows left on the rocks of Hiroshima. Together, the dark body and its empty crevices form a fragile unity, a Jungian fusion, whose only imbalance can be sickness or death.

In the iconography of a life, X-Ray plates are unwelcome guests in any photo-album, or box of portraits or holiday snaps. But the X-Ray is also a photograph, though of a poignant and particular kind. Like other photos it is only a fragment of a bigger story, only a rectangular slice of time, a split second in the trajectory of a life.

The writer Susan Sontag has noted the native surrealism of the photographic art, and how it relies on 'the very creation of a duplicate world, of a reality in the second degree, narrower but more dramatic than the one perceived by natural vision'. But in this novel reality, context is everything, and much of the meaning lies in the narrative. The tale told about the holiday snap surrounds it like a frame, and gives it a meaning. There in the telling is the feel of sunburnt skin, the full stomach, the mosquito bite, the sound of cicadas from behind the castle, the smells of the ocean or the scent of bougainvillaeas. But the story told of a radiograph, in square white hospital rooms, is sparse, and therefore mysterious: only a name, a date, a number, a diagnostic phrase, and always hovering somewhere in that room, an invisible human being.

But in other ways, X-Ray plates are a truer chronicle of the human moment. The random snap encapsulates the photographic past as well as the spectator's present, but the radiograph reveals more than just the biography of a body, and the labels given by the medical gaze. It is also a true photograph of the future, a snapshot of the skeleton inside waiting to be born, the one still hidden in its womb of flesh.

This parade of photographic skeletons and skulls, glowing on the screens of the radiology room, reminds me always of *El Día de los Muertos*, the Mexican fête of the dead. This is their All Souls' Day, an heir to the ancestor worship of the Aztecs, which takes place every autumn throughout Mexico. It is like a festival of the radiological eye. On this day skeletons of wood, plaster or papier-mâché are displayed, wearing bright everyday cloaks and sombreros, some carrying flowers, or wine, or musical instruments. Each is a *memento mori*, a grinning messenger to the plump and the unconcerned. In the early dawn light, families trek to the cemeteries, taking with them candles, tiny sweet skulls and skeleton candies, and ample offerings of flowers or food. They hold picnics near the graves of their relatives and, sitting on the ground, as one traveller has written, 'they tell and re-tell stories of the dear departed whose death they have come to mourn, and whose virtues they wish to perpetuate'. After the picnic the uneaten food is left at the gravesite, as a posthumous feast for the dead. For this one magical day, a singular hold in time, there is communion between the worlds of the living, and the worlds of the dead. The masks of life are stripped away, and the family members of both worlds share a meal across that transparent wall – thin as an X-Ray plate – that still divides them.

If you inject opaque dyes into the hollows and channels of your body, or drink them down deep into your crevices, then the white shapes on the X-Ray screen will paint a ghostly Rorschach inside your body.

For radiology reminds you that man is hollow. He is merely a doughnut, a bagel of flesh. You can outline the tortuous tunnel passing through this Hollow Man from his mouth down to his anus, with the creamy white liquid called Barium. Swallow a cupful, and as it waterfalls down the long tube of the oesophagus, you can see on the X-Ray screen some of the mythological possibilities of the human body.

There in the chest is the spinal column, with its twelve branching ribs, like a white Tree of Life in the centre of a Garden of Eden. In the lower part of the Garden, below the Tree, rest the two serpents of the bodily myth. The fat white worm of the Colon, its outline sketched in Barium, belches and stretches under the low hills of the diaphragm as small shudderings of peristalsis move the pellets of food along its length. And beneath it is the other serpent, the convoluted one, the Small Intestine, with its sluggish curves and crenellated back.

Elsewhere in the body, dye coursing through arteries and arterioles shows, as if from an aerial view, all the branching streams and tributaries of great, broad rivers flowing throughout the body. All the four rivers of Eden are there, Pison, Gihon, Hiddekel and Euphrates, with their forks and tributaries, their wandering brooks and tiny rivulets.

Now pour dye into the thick tubes that carry the vital air into the lungs, as they branch out from the windpipe into the 'bronchial tree'. See the ever-narrowing branches of this Tree of the Knowledge of Life fill with dye, and form a white and delicate bonsai, its feathery web of twigs and boughs bare for the winter. Notice how sometimes this tree carries on it a deadly fruit. The dye avoids an irregular area in the bonsai: instead of whiteness, there is a small black hole, a 'filling defect' on the film. A tumour has been found. Now a fatal Apple hangs from the branch, ready to poison the peace of the Garden.

[. . .]

Inject a dye into a vein in the arm, and the kidney excretes it into the urine. It flows through the two thin ureteric streams, from their stunted baobab openings in the kidney, down South to the pale oval lake of the bladder. In either direction, in the flanks of the Garden, a renal arteriogram reveals how in each kidney the blood vessels divide into an intricate tracery of tributaries – a Nile delta of tiny streams and rivers on either side of the body.

Here, in the newly transparent human form, an enigma repeats itself. Radiology has assembled the pieces of an ancient puzzle. The elements of the jigsaw, some old, some new, are all there on the screen: a shadowy Garden of rivers and hills, two Serpents, a white branching Tree of Life and one of Knowledge, a Cage, a line of Idols, and there – glowing in the very centre of the Garden – a lone pulsating Heart.

THIRTY-TWO

CARE MEASUREMENT

Niamh Merc

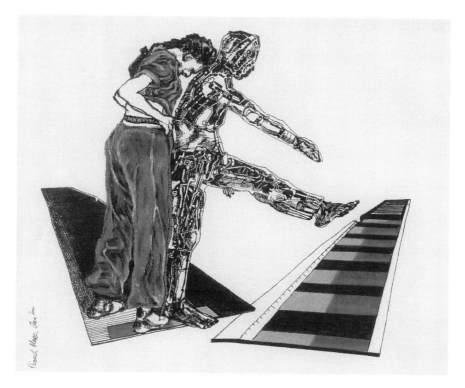

Measurement is a phenomenon that explores and puts an order onto our perception of our world. The compulsion to measure has affected both artists and scientists alike so that we gain in knowledge and perception of the world. The function of measurement in this image relies on both a physical assessment of ourselves (the woman) and a scientific assessment of the world we live in (the robot). My concern is that not enough attention/care is focused on the person within technological advancement, even though it strives to create a better world for the individual. In this age of technology, I feel that people have become somewhat distanced from a tactile and physical perception of themselves. In order to find a treatment, and to care for ourselves in a more holistic way, one needs to simultaneously measure in a scientific and corporeal manner by 'feeling' what our bodies are sensing so that we can find a balance between the physical and the psychological parts of ourselves. Virtual reality, while stimulating the imagination, has resulted in physical activities being forgotten about and becoming unused. One should try to be cautious not to lose one's own identity within the larger structure, and that is why the woman is taking care of her own well-being and is measuring herself in order to assess her own situation within this evolving world. Two roads, slightly overlapping, symbolize the past and the future. Both the robot and the person are moving towards a common direction and on to a future road.

THIRTY-THREE

'THE MEMORY BIRD': ACCOUNTS BY SURVIVORS OF SEXUAL ABUSE – EXTRACT 2

Emily Bird (1) and Runa Wolf (2)

1 A TRUE STORY ABOUT DREAMS

I am eight years old and I am standing in the school playing field. Other children look up at the sky with astonishment as a small aircraft circles lower and lower, until it is low enough to start unloading boxes which fall to the ground like Red Cross parcels. They are for me. I am not astonished because I have been waiting for them, but I had not really believed they would ever arrive. The other children watch in admiration as I start to open the boxes and reveal all the beautiful things that are just for me.

Shimmering beautiful dresses tumble out, covered with lace and jewels. Silk and velvet, singing pinks and kingfisher blues and golden yellows. And the jewels – bracelets, necklaces, tiaras; rubies, sapphires, emeralds, diamonds. Shawls and veils and shoes – oh, the shoes! Pink satin dancing shoes with pointed toes, embroidered with seed pearls – dozens and dozens of pairs. All this great richness and abundance for me, because at last I have been recognised and favoured, at last I am comforted and honoured. At last the hunger in my soul is filled.

This was my dream. I used it to comfort myself at night in bed when I was lonely and afraid, to help myself go to sleep. I never told anyone my fantasy because it would have shamed me to reveal my deprivation and my need; the deprivation which was seldom alleviated, the need that was so denied. I knew (but did not know) that I was different from other girls of my age, set apart and lonely. I felt it all through me but could not admit it to myself.

Source: Malone, C, Farthing, L, Marce, L. *The Memory Bird. Survivors of Sexual Abuse.* London: Virago Press, 1996. Reproduced by permission.

I had another dream too, which was also deeply comforting. In this one, I am playing with my best friend Sophy and we are climbing on the greenhouse. I accidentally slip and fall through the glass. I am cut all over and bleeding dangerously. Sophy, horrified, runs as fast as she can to get help; Sophy's father comes, and he carries me to the house and calls an ambulance. Sophy's mother bandages me. I have a broken leg too. Soon I am in hospital with my leg in plaster, and people around my bed, all worried about me and showing warm concern and anxiety for me. I do not imagine feeling any pain, but only a great relief that my wounds can be seen and attended to. I bask in the loving attention that I receive.

I *was* wounded, but the bleeding was inside. The crippling was inside. No one saw and no one comforted me.

I grew to be an adult and tried to live as though nothing was wrong inside me. But I was still crippled and still bleeding, and after a few years the anaesthetic of denial and amnesia began to wear off and I started to feel the pain of my wounds. Often it seemed intolerable. There were many times when I wished I was dead, just so that the pain would stop. I developed a new fantasy – different ways to commit suicide. The image I found most arresting was of myself lying dead in a bath filled with warm water, dressed in a long white gown, with swirls of blood curling around me from my opened veins. The classical Roman style. One night I dreamt that I saw a young dead girl in a bath filled with blood; in the same dream were babies impaled on long kitchen knives. Many of my sleeping dreams were filled with intruders, molesters, pursuers and other more graphic horrors.

Despite this, letting the pain through was the start of healing. It is nine years since I began to acknowledge my pain, to remember and recognise what had been done to me as a child, and to begin my recovery. Now I can talk about it and try to tell people how much it hurt, and still hurts. Often they do not want to hear. I am still lonely, and still hungry in my soul.

I am learning to dance. I started attending class once a week and gradually began to improve. My movements have become more and more fluid and graceful, my body more flexible and free. My confidence has grown; other people praise me. Sometimes I even feel beautiful. A woman in the class told me that my arm movements were so lovely that when she practised at home she tried to visualise my arms and copy the way I used them in dancing. One evening, the teacher asked the class to improvise to a piece of music which was slow and haunting and melodic; although Arabic, it had a Slavonic quality. The class danced, and when the music was over the teacher said 'I'm going to play it again, and I want you all to watch while Emily dances. This is Emily's music!'

I danced again. I felt the music as though it was coming from my body, and I danced my loneliness and my longing. When the music finished, I was astonished to see that my teacher had tears on her face. She came over to me and said 'That was beautiful!', and then she hugged me.

A part of my mind still refuses to believe that this really happened. It must have been a mistake, it was meant for someone else, it was a fluke and I will never be able to dance in the same way again ... but nevertheless, I have been asked to dance to that music at the concert. A part of me fears that I will stumble or fall or be graceless, but another part of me fears what might happen if I dance too well – who might be watching who will punish me if I reach too openly for beauty, for joy and for life?

But I am going to perform, and I am making a beautiful costume of shining gold and shimmering rainbow colours, covered in sequins and beads that sparkle like jewels.

When June comes, a lonely woman with lovely arms will step into the spotlight and dance.

2 WHOSE REALITY ARE YOU LIVING?

I first became interested in the difference between facts and the truth when writing autobiographical accounts of my experience of so-called mental illness. For me, 'recovery' was a process of redefining those experiences, rejecting the medical labels, and finding new words to express what I had been through. Coming to terms meant coming to my *own* terms, and thereby regaining some dignity and a sense of a continuous, rational self.

As I wrote, my accounts diverged more and more from my official medical case history. The facts were the same – dates of admission to hospital, numbers of ECT treatments, details of self-woundings, suicide attempts, a series of diagnoses – but the *truth* that I was searching for (you might say, creating for myself) involved some sort of *interpretation* of these facts, an *explanation* that assumed I had had a good reason for behaving the way I did.

What disturbed me most, during this process, was not the divergence of my account from that of the experts (others were also rejecting the experts at the time, even turning insanity into political rebellion or mystical enlightenment) but the way my *own* interpretation kept changing. Could I never fix the truth about my past? How many pasts could one person have? How could I tell which version (if any) was the true one?

But the real crisis came several years later, when I thought I had put the mental illness issues 'behind me'. Without realising it, I had for five or six years been hiding the full story of my past from others and minimising it in my own mind, in order to 'pass' as a fully functioning, if rather vulnerable, 'normal' member of society. Then I began to have nightmares about rape. At first, the dreams were of a man trying to break into my house, me frantically trying to bolt doors and windows, waking in terror just in time, before ... Increasingly, in this repeating scenario, there was a sickening sense that the man was someone I knew, and there would be a child in the house – my child – who I was terrified I would not be able to protect.

Then, in a particularly harrowing one, I was an amnesiac, fighting off the realisation that I had committed an unforgivable crime, one for which I would be boiled in oil. Then running, in nightclothes, through the streets, looking for my father to protect me, my father drawing me into his house for safety, my father sitting on my bed, my father . . . *the man I was trying to escape from.*

I had wondered before, when hearing survivors of sexual abuse describe their experiences, whether I too had been abused, but had dismissed this notion because I could not remember any such thing. I had always been frightened of my father, repulsed by him physically, and had had a difficult life, including a lot of problems with sexuality. But basically, I thought my parents, though inadequate in some ways, were decent people. I knew my problems originated in childhood, but blamed myself, and mental health professionals, for my having taken so long to 'get over' them.

When the nightmares had reached the pitch where I felt devastated for days after each one, I asked myself in earnest whether I could have been abused by my father. I went into a state of deep shock which lasted several months. Could it be true? I never doubted that the perpetrator, if there was one, was my father. Somehow I knew in my very bones that this whole issue was about him. I became obsessed with the idea, immobilised by it, haunted by it hour after hour. Eventually, worn out, I shelved the question, telling myself that if I had been abused it did not really matter. It was a long time ago, my parents were old now, and I would never know for sure . . .

But the idea returned with a vengeance exactly a year after the nightmares had begun, and this time I found the courage to follow it through. Breaking contact with my parents turned out to be the key to uncovering the truth. I could not open up the horror of my past while trying to hang on to the illusion of loving parents in the present.

Eventually I gave up my job to engage fully in the process of therapy. My parents, my brother, and for a time, my younger sister (who I know now was also abused) denied my 'disclosures', effectively rejecting me from the family. The almost overnight loss was devastating. In such a short time to lose my family, to have to reconstruct my whole personal history, to re-examine everything I thought I knew about the world, was overwhelming. I had no energy left for anything else. I was swamped by grief. The rage came later. And finally, much later – excitement, transformation, triumph, calm.

So now I have this new version of my past. I still have no clear-cut memories, no visual information, nothing verifiable from the outside. Yet I *know* I was abused. Apart from my family, those who know me have never doubted me. I have relived the abuse, horrifically, many times in therapy. I remember it physically and emotionally, if not visually, and that is good enough for me.

It explains everything – my bizarre sexual awareness from early child-hood, my gender-identity confusion, desperate sexual experiences with men, acts of self-mutilation, the so-called mental illness – it makes sense of my past in a way no other 'interpretation' has done.

But what does all this imply about what is real, about how we arrive at the truth? My parents and my Anglican vicar brother still vehemently deny my allegations. I have no proof, other than the evidence of my life's experi-ences, my emotions, my dreams, my body-memories – in other words, my *self*, my sense of *who I am*. These things, which are everything to me – my integrity, my humanity – are they, in the face of a lack of hard evidence, enough?

Not for a court of law. Not for those who prefer to think that parents, simply by virtue of being parents, have some greater access to reality than their offspring. Not for those experts who have manufactured the false-memory syndrome and concocted, like witch-hunters of the past, a con-spiracy of therapists out to bring the family to its knees.

But my own truth is more than good enough for me. There is a choice. Not to believe in my self means I am either a vicious liar, a complete fool, or mentally ill. I know I am none of these. And since I placed my trust firmly in my own version of the past, my present world has changed. In place of an isolated alienhood, a toehold in the normal world I wanted so badly to accept me, I have both feet firmly planted and am much taller and infinitely more capable than I realised.

So have I fixed the truth about my past now, written the definitive life-story? I am sure I have not. My past will continue to change as my under-standing of my self continues to grow. Maybe more memories of abuse will return, maybe other aspects of my childhood will assume greater significance. But this prospect no longer worries me. What I know now is that facts (dates, witnessed events, evidence that will stand up in court) are no more related to the truth than a railway timetable is to the experience of a journey.

The past that matters is not 'out there' but inside of me, my inner reality, the foundation of the me that I experience in the present, and project into the future. This inner reality is a dynamic, creative process, not an object which can be pinned down, trapped in time to form a single eternal truth. Trusting this process liberates creative powers and sharpens perception. It is not a hazy, anything-goes, believe-what-you-like fantasy world, but a gathering of the senses, the intellect, the intuition into one powerful focus of awareness – it is being 'I', the author of my own exist-ence, furnishing my world with the meanings and values which I have carefully chosen. It is being alive, it is being human in the profoundest sense. Anything less is a self-mutilation, however subtle or invisible.

I believe now that 'the truth' is always a personal choice, an act of faith – no less for my parents or the false-memory experts than for me. You have to decide, to make a commitment. Will you believe the denying parents who claim that simply because they were the grown-ups at the time they must be telling the truth now? (Because parents inevitably define the world for us when we are dependent children, do they still have the right to do so when we are grown?) Will you put your trust in 'facts', in the sort of evidence that law courts demand, in psychological theories about memory based on scientific research? Or will you dare to listen to the truth embodied in a nightmare, to accept the evidence of an adult body in the throes of a remembered rape, to recognise the logic of a reconstructed life-story, to trust that deep intuitive knowledge, that gut conviction of what is right?

It's a frightening, risky business. Our culture has a very limited idea of what counts as real, has vested the power to define reality in a masculine minority for whom 'science', the experts, are often the spokespeople, the PR merchants. They will always have an answer – a new syndrome or complex, backed up by research, statistics, evidence – to every challenge to their monopoly on reality. It's no good waiting for 'the truth' about childhood sexual abuse to be untangled 'out there', or for your own memory to provide a neatly packaged set of facts which at last no one will be able to dispute. When it comes to the fabric of our own lives, the basis of our identity, our Selves, we have to be our own experts. We each of us have to decide how to recognise the truth, how to define and name reality. At the heart of the question 'what is true?' is the more fundamental issue: whose side are you on?

THIRTY-FOUR

EXTRACT FROM 'THE OFFICERS' WARD'

Marc Dugain

Louis Levauchelle had joined us in November 1915. His wound was very similar to mine and to those of several other wounded men on our floor. A hole in the middle of the face, as if the flesh had been sucked in from the inside. He had already undergone three attempted grafts, in hospitals with less of a reputation than ours, first with the cartilage of a pig, then a sow, then a calf. All three rejected.

He kept photographs of his wife and two sons by his bedside, photographs that had stayed with him through all the fourteen months of fighting. Levauchelle often made up a fourth at *belote*.

During the early months of the war, the military hierarchy had encouraged men with maxillofacial wounds to stay in their hospitals, even when their condition allowed them to go out. The open display of our wounds might have been a blow to the morale of a nation waging a war which was no closer to an end and which demanded a growing commitment. Visits were authorised sparingly and took place in a room on the ground floor that resembled a classroom in a Parisian secondary school on examination day, with two desks and four chairs.

Levauchelle wrote often to his family, but like the rest of us, he had never had the courage to admit how serious his condition was.

His first visit from his wife and children took place on 21 June 1916, the first day of summer.

That morning, Levauchelle asked our advice as to what day clothes would be most appropriate. He hesitated between keeping his bandages

Source: Dugain, M. *The Officers' Ward*. London: The Orion Publishing Group Ltd, 2000.
Reproduced by permission.

on, wearing a black headband, and simply leaving his wounds exposed. I recommended the headband, thinking that it would be the least upsetting. He was as agitated as a child.

I can still see his tall figure coming back along the corridor to the ward after the visit. When he saw me, he collapsed on my shoulder, in no state even to speak. He dropped onto his bed, and Weil and I stood by him, powerless to do anything, until night fell. When the lights were turned out, we left him.

The next morning, knowing from experience that the moment of waking was the most difficult time to get through, I got up and approached his bed. If I had not lost my sense of smell, the odour of spilled blood would have alerted me. He had taken his own life.

The day before, he had asked a nurse to buy him a packet of sweets for his children. As she felt he might be unsteady on his feet, she had suggested she accompany him to the visiting room.

Neither his wife nor his children had recognised him. The elder of the two boys had run off down the corridor, screaming: 'Not my daddy! Not my daddy!' His wife had taken the children by the hand, promising to come back when he was more 'himself'.

A mass was said for Louis in the hospital chapel. Four of his ward companions, those whose sense of balance had not been affected by their wounds, took part. The priest officiated in a monotonous voice – he must have been performing one funeral service after another for many months on end.

I learned from Penanster that it had taken him a long time to persuade the priest to say mass for a suicide. In the middle of the service, Marguerite appeared, a tall figure with her face concealed behind a scarf, and knelt in the back row.

At the end of the service, we all came out together. Penanster, who was in front, stopped in the corridor that led back to the wards, turned and made us swear with him that none of us would take his own life. The body was taken away to be buried in a place called Marnes-la-Coquette. Sometimes, the name of a place is quite inappropriate to the circumstances.

Weil suggested that we should ask for permission to go out on 14 July. I was not keen on the idea, but Penanster agreed that it was time to confront the world. For Marguerite, it was still much too early.

We debated for a while what to wear, and finally decided to go out in uniform and head bandages. I had managed to retrieve my own uniform. By some miracle, it had reached the hospital laundry, and when it was returned to me it was spotless – I had expected to find it as disfigured as I was. Penanster borrowed a uniform from a cavalry officer on the first floor. Weil could not lay his hands on an aviator's uniform, and finally squeezed into that of an infantry lieutenant. The sleeves of his tunic only reached as far as mid-arm, and his trousers barely covered his socks.

Our 'lost squadron' set off about eleven in the morning. I don't recall ever in my life having known such intense fear. Even before the most major operations, I had never felt such anguish, or been so dizzy. It was as if I had been asked to cross Paris jumping from one roof to another.

We headed towards the Seine, Penanster in front, head held high, easily the most presentable of the three of us. Then came Weil, looking straight ahead. I brought up the rear, my eyes on the ground, staring intently at the manhole covers.

The sky was a faded blue, with high clouds scurrying in the wind.

An old man coming home from his morning constitutional stopped on the doorstep of his building, looked us slowly up and down, one after the other, and raised his hat to salute us.

The fresh air bothered me – I had never before realised there could be so much of it. Like anything of which there is a surfeit, it soon became oppressive.

Paris seemed deserted. There were just a few women and old people about. It was as if the whole country had emigrated.

Fifty metres away, and heading straight for us, was a whole herd of children led by a young blonde woman. It was time to turn back. I tugged at my friends' sleeves. But Weil was determined to buy himself a croissant. We tried our best to explain to him that bread was already becoming scarce, but he was adamant. It was as if he wanted to give our excursion a purpose. We spotted a bakery on the corner of the boulevard. The window was empty. There was a woman inside, polishing the display shelf, with her back to us. Weil entered the shop first, with us hard on his heels, like carriages attached to a locomotive. The woman turned. Her eyes opened wide, and she dropped her cloth and a loaf of black bread she had been holding in her other hand. The loaf rolled along the floor and stopped at Weil's feet. Without giving him time to pick it up, the woman rushed to seize her merchandise, as if snatching her child from the hands of a stranger. The loaf nestling in her arms, she retreated behind the counter. Pretending to ignore her terror, Penanster stepped forward.

'Three croissants, please,' he asked her, very politely. 'Croissants?' she replied. 'Croissants? You must be joking! All I have is two loaves of black bread, and they're already sold.' She stared at us with an air of finality. 'You're not Germans, by any chance?'

Weil burst into loud laughter, and we turned on our heels and left. My whole body was shaking, as if it were suddenly the middle of winter. I begged my friends to go back, and Penanster and Weil concurred.

When, some time later, I suggested they go out again without me, they proposed a game of cards instead, making the excuse that I had fleeced them the day before.

We never again mentioned that disastrous outing.

THIRTY-FIVE

CARE IN THE COMMUNITY

Jennifer Hockey

Pick up your pads Dad, pick up your blanket.
Get in the car 'cos you can't stay alone.
Get on the road now, get your belongings.
Come up with us and you'll soon feel at home.

Where am I going? Where am I staying?
Where are my house keys?
Where am I sleeping?

Beverley, Yorkshire; Beverley, Yorkshire.
West of Wetwang, south of Sledmere.
North of Newbald, east of Eden.

How can I travel when I've no money?
How will I get home
Safely to Fore Street?

Nevermore, Daddy.
Nevermore Fore Street.
Nevermore home, now you've spent up your years.
Beverley, Yorkshire; Beverley, Yorkshire.
Only one way out of
Beverley, Yorkshire.

THIRTY-SIX

LIVING WITH A DEADLY DISEASE

Anonymous

Shortly after the birth of her second child, Meg was diagnosed with rheumatoid arthritis. As the disease progressed she was given a further diagnosis of systemic lupus erythematosus. Lupus, as it is most commonly called, is a potentially dangerous chronic auto-immune disease that can affect virtually any organ of the body. In lupus, the immune system that normally protects the body becomes hyperactive, and forms antibodies that attack healthy tissues and organs including the skin, joints, kidneys, brain, lungs, heart and blood. For Meg the condition was serious and she slowly deteriorated and eventually died at the age of 54.

What follows is Meg's account of living with that experience and the way in which she began to experience her body as something separate that needed to be monitored because it could let her down at any moment. Meg is not her real name.

'When I wake up the first thing I ask myself is "How do I feel?" I move my legs and then my arms very slowly to feel how much pain there is. My husband will have left me a cold drink to take my tablets with and so I sit up slowly and take my pills and then wait for about 20 minutes for the tablets to work and start to get up. Just lately I have felt increasingly tired – I can't really explain it – but it just drags me down and makes me feel lousy. The awful thing is that when I go to bed and lie down I just become more aware of how uncomfortable I am and so I end up taking sleeping tablets to help me to sleep and I don't think that they help. I don't think that it's a proper sleep.

On a good day I can go and shower and be ready within the hour – but if I feel unwell – or if my head is really bad – then I just have a wash and start the dialysis. I have to do this four times a day. I empty one load of fluid from my abdomen through one tube and then fill it through another tube with new fluid and empty it about four hours later. I do this every four hours and I always have this abdomen full of fluid – it's like always being pregnant.

It takes me ages to do anything partly because I am so out of breath and partly because I seem to hurt all over – especially in my joints – I've got walking sticks but my wrists are so weak that they are not easy to use. Some days I feel much better and I want to skip around the room – but most days now I feel awful. I feel angry at this lupus. I feel that my body has let me down. I've got to the point where I hate this body – it is as if I am a prisoner and trapped inside it. There is so much I want to do – there are so many things that I want to see and now I can't do or see any of them.

I wouldn't mind if I could just be at home but in the last two years I have spent nearly half of that time in hospital. I was in there for 12 weeks before Christmas when I broke my hip. I just stepped off the pavement and I felt it go. I had to stay in hospital and have a hip replacement. My spine is crumbling and I've had several crush fractures – not that anyone can do anything for that. Then my kidneys failed and the dialysis meant that I had to have this fistula made to provide permanent access for the dialysis – so that I could do it at home. I just dread what might happen next. Every time I feel something different happening – I think "Oh, no! What's going on now?" When I was taking the chemotherapy tablets I had the most horrendous nightmares. I can't describe how horrid they were. I am sure that it was the treatment destroying my body and my mind was warning me that I was in terrible danger.

I can't make any plans – I never know how I will feel. I live for my children now – all that I look forward to is seeing them and hearing about their life. I want them to have what I couldn't have.'

PART IV

DIFFICULT ENCOUNTERS

INTRODUCTION

Caroline Malone

This part of the book deals with encounters and relationships which could be described as difficult both by health and social care professionals and by people who receive services. Times of extreme stress can challenge effective communication. The accounts in this part of the book explore these issues by using personal reflections. Examples include such experiences as breaking news of a terminal illness, looking after a dying child, dealing with a traumatic event such as rape or sectioning someone with mental illness. A variety of accounts from different perspectives highlight the impact that each form or manner of communication had on the person experiencing difficulty or trauma. Some of them show very clearly how poor communication can lead to poor or inadequate care.

Some accounts are from the service user's perspective and give insights into what is perceived as helpful or unhelpful by them and by their carers. Alexander Stuart and Ann Totterdell describe the different encounters they experience in caring for their terminally ill child, all of them difficult but not all supportive. Alex describes how a junior doctor broke the news that the cancer was untreatable in front of his son and was impervious to their attempts to silence him, saying that the child would not understand. The parents' shock was confused with their anger over his behaviour and made it impossible for them to take in the information and ask relevant questions.

The author of 'September 11th: a professional victim' describes her responses to different professional interventions after being raped, some of which were supportive and some very difficult for her. She has the added insights from her own work as a professional adding another dimension to her experiences.

In the third selection of accounts from *The Memory Bird* we hear the voices of people who have experienced extreme trauma and sought help from the mental health services – some angry and some clearly stating what they needed but also how effective the appropriate help could be. These are also examples of how people's responses to breakdowns in communication can result in behaviour being wrongly

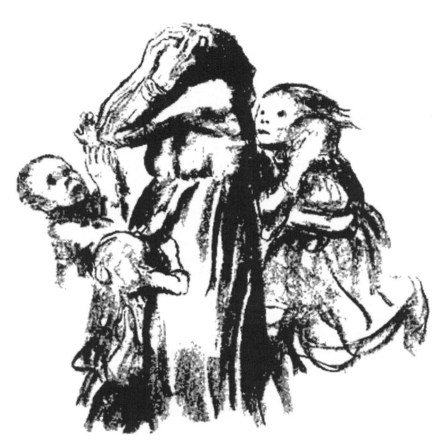

Times of extreme stress can challenge effective communication. Such experiences as breaking news of a terminal illness, looking after a dying child, dealing with a traumatic event such as rape or sectioning someone with mental illness can challenge the skills and resources of professionals and carers to their limits. (Illustration reproduced from a drawing by Käthe Kollwitz entitled 'Killed in action' (1921), © DACS, 2004.)

interpreted and labelled, creating further problems. For example, in her poem, 'Abuse: the power of articulating experiences' Alex Benjamin describes how people become labelled as difficult when they express anger or distress. In 'Ghosts in the machine' in Part V, Charis Alland describes how misunderstandings lead to the dissemination of inaccurate information about her, which can then become almost impossible to correct.

The section also contains passages from professionals and talks about the pressures they experience. In 'The junior doctor on the sweaty horrors of a mental health tribunal' Michael Foxton clearly expresses how painful it can be for practitioners when people are sectioned. He wryly comments on the process of repeatedly rebuilding his relationships. The field notes by Jane Seymour in 'Reproducing subjectivity and meaning in nursing work' demonstrate the emotional costs of decision-making and the process of trying to make a difference in caring for a dying person in particularly difficult circumstances when the nurse she is talking to breaks down and starts to cry. It shows clearly the importance of providing support for professionals in extreme situations.

In the article by Michele Hanson, Nell Dunn expresses a great deal of empathy for professionals by looking at her own difficulties as a carer and talks about the unreasonable expectations that society has of people working in the health and care sectors. Dunn is opposed to 'doctor bashing' and feels the expectations we have of doctors are often unrealistic: *'We're expecting doctors to have a depth of kindness that I certainly haven't got,'* she says. *'I'm impatient, irritable, forgetful, but they must be tremendously intelligent, generous and never forget anything.'* This article also recalls the accounts in Part I, bringing out how expectations of professionals have changed over time from a model of paternalism and grateful deference, to one where professionals are expected to respond to demand, be open and accountable, and provide quality and choice under conditions that are often extremely stressful for them. The extract from 'The Brothers Karamazov' gives us a very sharp insight into one aspect of the motivation of those choosing to serve others and the way reality may blunt the edge of the initial idealism.

Underlying these accounts are many different assumptions: the form of communication is vitally important and has an enormous impact on the way users or carers cope with their illness or trauma; effective communication involves skills which can be developed and power imbalances can create problems and are more apparent in the changing climate in the health and care sectors. Service users stress the importance of empathy, respect and clarity in communication while the professionals' emphasis is on the barriers that can be created by competing demands. Oliver Sacks describes how dramatically his ability to cope with his illness was affected by his various interactions with different professionals. The need to maintain channels of communication is also seen as vital. Oliver Sacks describes being overwhelmed with despair when he feels no one is listening to him. He relates how easily this can happen and how critical the responses of the professionals can be. It seems that all the power rests with them, making the service user feel very vulnerable.

What comes through very clearly is the role communication plays in the effectiveness of care. Again and again those receiving care express the importance of empathy and positive regard. The need to listen, the need to be sensitive and the willingness to overcome barriers becomes more critical in extreme circumstances, especially where there are additional difficulties such as language or culture. The interpreter's perspective in 'Going the extra mile' shows the pain and humiliation that a failure to act sensitively can cause in working with diverse cultures and languages, and in 'The sound barrier', Michael Simmons talks about what it feels like to be deaf, quoting some words he had read, which 'brought tears of understanding to my eyes':

> When you impatiently say 'Never mind'
> I shrivel up inside
> For I frantically fought to hear what you said
> And you don't even know I tried.

In 'Text Appeal' Charis Alland writes about the importance of finding alternative methods of communicating when more obvious channels are blocked due to illness or environment. This is also vividly described by Jean-Dominique Bauby in the extract from 'The Diving-Bell and the Butterfly' in Part III. Both are cut off from the outside world by their illness, one being a state of depression and the other a physical condition, but both describe the vital importance of maintaining channels of communication. Bauby talks about the importance of maintaining a level of anger and resentment as a safety valve, to keep his mind sharp and avoid becoming indifferent.

Communication is also a way of keeping safe. If you cannot communicate you are vulnerable. An extreme example of this is where abuse takes place because the victim is unable to speak out, as the author of 'I mustn't tell anyone. But he did hurt me, mum' explains when talking about the rape of a woman with a learning disability. The perpetrator was able to control her because she was unable to understand what was happening, believed his threats and could not defend herself. The abuse was only discovered by accident.

Times of extreme stress can heighten the need for communication to be effective and challenge the people involved to be aware and sensitive of what their words and attitudes convey. The accounts in this part of the book explore these issues by using some very evocative personal reflections.

THIRTY-SEVEN

THE JUNIOR DOCTOR ON THE SWEATY HORRORS OF A MENTAL HEALTH TRIBUNAL

Michael Foxton

'You're a shit doctor who never listens and I'll be out of here by lunchtime.' I had almost forgotten it was Nigel's tribunal today. We were getting on pretty well until today, but I guess his solicitor has been in talking to him. That means we won't be friends for a while, and he will be refusing his medication for at least a week. I try and smile warmly until I remember how paranoid that makes him.

I hate sectioning people. Nigel had to be sectioned because he was going around telling everyone in his council block that they should stop selling crack to their children. He didn't start getting beaten up until he suggested to the parents that they should hand the children over into his care, where he could give them the love they need. It was all very well meant, but you just have to try and work around the fact that people get angry about that kind of thing in the middle of the night.

We all trundle through the corridors to the conference room. Nigel stands, with his solicitor, staring at me. I stand with the nurse and the social worker. The tribunal keeps us waiting for half an hour, until we are called in by the clerk.

They all have cups of coffee, and neat little china plates with biscuits on them. The barrister who is chairing the hearing addresses everyone by their formal title, and we sit on opposite sides of the table: everyone has an expensive leather documents folder, except for me and Nigel. I feel deeply out of place, and very worried.

'Dr Foxton, are you satisfied that the patient has a mental illness, dis-

Source: *Guardian* 14 January 2003. Reproduced by permission.

order, or impairment; and that it is of a nature and degree such as to justify detention under the Mental Health Act 1983?'

Umm. 'Yes,' I reply. Confidently.

'Yes, what?' I look around.

'Yes, your honour?' I smile weakly and start to sweat. Taking my jumper off would look really bad right now.

The tribunal doctor looks over warmly. He is about 70, clearly retired, and being paid by the hour. 'When the chair asks you that question, he means: which of the three is it, and under the terms of the Mental Health Act, is it nature, or degree, or both?' I look up at him, willing him to help me out some more. 'You have to say which, now.'

The chair casts him an evil look. He smiles warmly. 'Umm. Illness.' I flounder. 'And, well, nature and degree, please.'

I had never really thought about it. I blush again. Nigel looks baffled, and delighted. The barrister just looks angry and rich.

Nigel's solicitor rounds on me and makes me go through my report. I have to recount, in front of Nigel, all his psychiatric symptoms, in the most technical medical language, because this is a formal legal hearing. It feels as if I am accusing him of a crime: you are charged with stopping taking your medication at home, and hearing voices, and that those voices did compel you to behave very strangely; you are charged with getting into a squabble on a crowded ward with a nasty character over cigarettes, where your understandable misunderstanding of her mental health problems led you to get into a nasty argument and you both being sedated and secluded.

It would feel massively trite and completely counterproductive to mention that he is incredibly charming and funny, and that his delusions and hallucinations are so painfully understandable, in the context of his shit life, that you sometimes feel like giving him a big hug and trying to explain it all as best you can. Either way, after I read out the list of charges, he will probably never tell me about a single symptom ever again for as long as he lives.

Nigel keeps interrupting to deny these episodes. His solicitor pulls my report apart, implying that I am some kind of sinister jailer.

I think back to our teaching: tribunals are supposed to be inquisitorial, not adversarial. We are supposed to get together and work out what is best. These guys all want to be on Judge Judy. They grill me for an hour, even though there is no way in a million years anyone would let Nigel out of hospital until the medication starts to kick in and gets him back to his normal self. When we start discussing his insight, I deliver what now feels like my trump card – and that thought makes me realise I have sunk to their level.

'He told me, yesterday, that if he got off at the tribunal he would leave hospital immediately and stop taking the tablets.' QED.

'I never,' he shouts. The tribunal retire to consider. But everyone knew the verdict before we even started. The lawyers are a few pounds richer, and a few inches taller; and Nigel and I will have to start from square one all over again.

THIRTY-EIGHT

EXTRACTS FROM 'THE SHORT LIFE AND DEATH OF JOE BUFFALO STUART', INCLUDING WIGGLY WORM

Alexander Stuart and Ann Totterdell

These extracts are from the moving account of a small boy's illness and death jointly told by his parents, Alex and Ann.

Alex: Your whole life can change in so few seconds. The whole of Sunday evening became like a dream – too numbing to call a nightmare – but two particular moments stand out as the points at which our lives shifted from what had seemed like normality into a world of extremes: extreme love and extreme fear.

The first was when Lucy Moore pointed out Joe's swollen left kidney. My immediate thought was, 'Dialysis!' In a fraction of a second, my son, whom I loved more than anything in the world, went from being a healthy child to someone who might have to spend the rest of his life taking extra care and making regular visits to hospitals.

But more than this, I was thrown back to a memory from my childhood: a school-friend's father had died from kidney failure. Already, before the word 'cancer' had been mentioned by anyone, I was scared enough about the prospects for Joe if he were to be left with only one kidney.

The other moment, of course, which changed everything was when Lilias Lamont told us, with a degree of certainty which unnerved me, that she thought it might be cancer.

Source: Stuart, A, Totterdell, A. *The Short Life and Death of Joe Buffalo Stuart*. London: Vintage, 1990. Reproduced by permission of Penguin Group (UK).

We had just met her. I had no clear idea what a registrar was; only later did I learn that she was senior to the house officers and, in fact, next in line under the consultant. I remember her manner at that moment, which was a mixture of cautious and direct. If she was fairly sure of the diagnosis, she was less than certain how to tell us. I remember her hair, which fell forward on to her face at the sides. I remember her glasses, the unhappy line of her mouth as she tried to make her words matter-of-fact rather than alarming: 'I expect you've already thought about the possibility that it might be cancer.'
[. . .]

Cancer meant death to me. The only possible outcome in my mind at that moment was death. I thought Joe might be dead within the week, I literally thought that it might all be over within a matter of days, and yet, only two and a half or three hours ago, we had brought Joe to the hospital with what we thought was a bad stomach-ache. We were meant to be at my sister's soon for dinner.

In this sense, I think we were lucky to be told so quickly. You hear so often of bad diagnoses, of long periods of doubt and uncertainty when doctors aren't sure or simply make mistakes. Of course, a mistake might have been made here, and despite the hell it put us through, we would gladly have heard that it wasn't cancer after all. But we were grateful for how promptly and straightforwardly we were told, and if Lilias's choice of words hardly seemed adequate, I don't envy her the fact that she had to tell us at all. How do you tell anyone that their child has cancer? I would far rather have heard that I had it myself.

I know now that Ann's immediate reaction was different from mine, in terms of the shape of her fear. Her first husband had died of lung cancer; her father had also died of cancer. She knew the pattern it could follow, the months of treatment, the slow and possibly painful decline. She was afraid of a long, drawn-out period of suffering for Joe. I was afraid that I would lose him within a week.
[. . .]

Ann: The most immediate problem after the diagnosis was, what were we going to tell Joe? He was about to have a major operation, something completely outside his experience. The tangible parts would be the pre-med, the anaesthetic, bandages and, most in need of explanation, a lot of pain afterwards. Somehow we had to justify all this to him, and give him a picture of what was going to happen, as simply as possible and without frightening him. The concept of a bug was one he was familiar with from various minor ailments, so we told him that there was a bug in his tummy that was making it hurt, and that the doctors were going to get rid of it with what was called an operation.
[. . .]

I felt comfortable about telling him this because, as far as the surgery was concerned, it was true. A more complicated outcome was still hypothetical. It's hard now to think that though our imaginations turned this into a threatening period, it was also the time when we were being reassured that the survival rate from a Wilms was over 90 per cent. Our favourite house officer described it to us as 'a lazy old tumour' which rarely had secondaries.

[. . .]

Ann: On Wednesday we finally heard the results of the histology. Since we'd learnt that there were cells in Joe's bone marrow, the overall picture had become disturbing, but there was still the image of a Wilms as a passive type of cancer, suggesting one easily treated, to reassure us.

I suppose Dr Phillips, Joe's oncologist, and Dr Sinclair, the ward's consultant, were unavailable that day, because a junior member of Dr Phillips's staff, Dr Peck, arrived in Joe's room to talk to us. Although Joe was awake he launched into an explanation of how the histology had shown that Joe had a very rare, untreatable type of tumour cell.

The shock this announcement brought was on two levels: the mere fact of what he was saying; and that he was saying it in front of Joe with no consideration for how Joe would interpret what was being said or how his parents were reacting to it. I had to break away from the conversation to distract Joe. Maybe Dr Peck thought it was an expression of indifference, because he came over to Joe's cot to attempt to explain it all to me. I was gripped by panic at what he was telling us, and by an urgent need to stop him speaking in front of Joe. As I steered the doctor towards the door, I hissed that I didn't want to discuss it in Joe's hearing. 'It's all right, he won't understand,' was his reaction.

Even now when I think of that day, the shock of what he was telling us is confused with anger at what we felt and still feel was his appalling mismanagement of the situation. His apparent lack of forethought created a climate in which we were unable to absorb and ask questions calmly about what he was telling us.

[. . .]

We sensed at times that the hospitals were straining at the seams to maintain their patient care, and that their ability to cope was very much due to the determination of the staff to compensate for shortcomings elsewhere. Joe was never denied any treatment due to cut-backs, but we were acutely aware of the nightly telephone checks on bed availability at other hospitals and the fact that on some nights in London there were virtually no spare paediatric beds available in the event of an emergency.

We felt immensely grateful to the NHS for providing total care for Joe, as our right, at a time when the last thing we needed was the anxiety of wondering how we would pay for expensive, long-term medical treatments. Simply deciding whether to subject him to the rigours of those treatments was painful enough without taking cost into account, and the experience reinforced in me – not simply because of Joe, but through watching other, less advantaged families on various wards – an absolute belief that public medicine is the only fair and humane way of providing health care in a society. [. . .]

[WIGGLY WORM]

Ann: The pattern of Joe's treatment continued much as before, even though we had moved. Before we made a final decision about Brighton, we had asked if Joe could remain a patient at St Stephen's. The answer was yes. We had been reluctant to change hospitals when he was in the middle of being treated by people completely familiar with his condition and in whom we had developed a great deal of trust, and for similar reasons Dr Sinclair and Dr Phillips were equally reluctant to hand him over to new doctors. Dr Sinclair immediately offered to make contact with the children's hospital in Brighton, the Royal Alexandra, so that Joe's weekly blood tests could be carried out there; and, since the hospital had a cancer ward, Joe would have contact with experienced staff.

We felt a little embarrassed at the role the Royal Alexandra was forced to play in our lives: the Cinderella hospital that did the boring blood tests while St Stephen's kept control of the interesting facets of Joe's treatment. But as far as continuity and Joe's sense of security with his existing doctors were concerned, it made sense. Given the way that all medical staff – doctors, nurses, technicians, physiotherapists – tend to circulate in search of promotion or experience, there is no realistic basis for assuming that London hospitals are better than provincial ones, yet to two London chauvinists, our first visit to the Royal Alexandra was an unfortunate confirmation of all our fears.

From the moment Joe arrived on the ward for his first blood test, he was bombarded with a flood of baby talk he had never experienced before. His Hickman line, which he always called his line, was constantly referred to as a wiggly worm, or his wiggly, a bit of tweeness he found quite incomprehensible. Apparently wiggly worms weren't flushed in the way Joe was used to; they had 'big drinks'.

We had always believed that children are quite capable of using a proper vocabulary and that, in the case of the Hickman line, giving its correct name and explaining its function was a good deal more helpful in demystifying it than any amount of cute language. At the time the line had been installed Joe was not particularly articulate, and yet he had understood perfectly what it was for, and had been justly proud of his mastery of the medical jargon.

Now, in a children's hospital, on a cancer ward, where if anything we should be dealing with more enlightened people, we found ourselves having to translate bewildering euphemisms back into normal English. Once Joe had cracked their code he dealt with the matter himself. 'You mean my line,' he would say if anyone mentioned a wiggly worm. On one occasion, when he was a bit older, he stunned a nurse who'd been foolish enough to talk about 'a big drink of salty water' by saying reprovingly that he hoped she meant saline, because he didn't want sea water in his line.

All of this may reflect personalities more than medical expertise, but

Alex and I were a little disconcerted by the attitudes we encountered even over the simple matter of a blood test. At that time Joe's Hickman line had developed a leak and had been repaired, and no longer gave blood so reliably. On the occasions when blood wouldn't come at the first attempt, the staff at the Royal Alexandra wanted to resort to a needle immediately, causing Joe great distress, which seemed out of keeping with people used to caring for very sick children. With patience the line would always yield blood, and yet that patience, not an expendable luxury even in an overworked department, but an absolute essential in treating an apprehensive child, was frequently lacking. Our early impression of the cancer ward at the Royal Alexandra was of a staff perhaps understandably desensitized by constant contact with terminally ill children.

The first impression was, of course, far too simplistic, and in due course we became aware of the department's many virtues, as well as its failings. In particular, they demystified our approach to Joe's bouts of neutropenia, giving us the confidence to keep him at home instead of admitting him to St Stephen's for reverse barrier nursing. They also taught us to maintain his Hickman line ourselves, a simple task made complicated by the need for minute attention to sterile procedures, but which was liberating in reducing our dependence on hospitals.

In other words, it was probably no better or worse than any other ward in any other hospital, but our first crucial impressions were unfavourable, and we were constantly thankful that St Stephen's, where everyone had always made us feel that Joe was as special to them as he was to us, still wanted to care for him. [. . .]
[. . .]

For now, physiotherapy was the most important treatment for Joe. Though he had made such encouraging progress at Charing Cross [St Stephen's], and some movement was coming back into his feet, he had a long way to go. [. . .] On our first afternoon we were introduced to Linda Williams, who was to take charge of Joe's physiotherapy. The arrival of Linda into Joe's life was a huge milestone. Not only did she prove to be brilliant at her job, but she had the authority to make Joe work when he didn't really want to. She was like the best teacher in the world, sympathetic and kind, but firm and determined to keep the upper hand. The interesting thing was that Joe, who was very good at controlling people, loved it, and he loved her.
[. . .]

When Alex telephoned the ward to report that Joe was in pain again, he assumed that Joe would be X-rayed to find out the source of the trouble. 'What's the point?' was the response of the staff nurse he spoke to. Her attitude made us tense and uneasy. We had been told by Dr Cree during our initial conversation that Joe would have more radiotherapy if he needed it, and an X-ray would be the first step towards this.
[. . .]

Dr Cree's [at Royal Alexandra] attitude, which seemed to us to consist of letting Joe get to the brink of paralysis before any action was taken, combined with the nurse's remark, made us very dissatisfied and insecure. Suddenly we began to feel as if Joe were some laboratory specimen they were watching. The atmosphere was becoming less sympathetic, as if Joe had been written off.

During the next few days this feeling was reinforced a couple of times. Once, when I rang to ask for more codeine for Joe, which was always prescribed by Dr Cree and obtained from the hospital pharmacy, the staff nurse I spoke to asked in a very offhand way why I couldn't get it from Joe's GP. As our GP had no involvement in his treatment, and getting prescriptions from her would be a good deal more complicated and time-consuming, I viewed this remark with some mistrust. It seemed like another sign of dismissal.

In the same period, when I had taken Joe to the Hospital with me to collect a prescription, I mentioned to another staff nurse the possibility of an X-ray for Joe as he was still in pain. In front of Joe she said coolly, 'What's the point?' This phrase was becoming too familiar and once more I felt the chill of abandonment. 'Dr Cree did say Joe might have some radiotherapy if his pain got worse,' I told her firmly. To her credit, when she heard this, the nurse immediately went to speak to Dr Cree and came back and offered to look after Joe while I saw her.

I went into Dr Cree's office and told her how desperate we were, how the pain seemed to be getting worse, and our greatest fear was that Joe would be paralysed again. She explained that the tumour was in a completely different site and that, though it could be incapacitating, its effect would not be as dramatic as the first tumour last April. There was a shred of reassurance in this, but it still seemed to me in my demoralized state a harsh and over-clinical response. The wait-and-see policy still stood.

I began to think that the Royal Alexandra was a very bad place for Joe. I felt he was surrounded by people infected by a brutal, and to us incomprehensible, attitude. Perhaps by failing to get well he had become unimportant – the idea of throwing more pain-killers at him, while tumours which might be controlled were destroying him, seemed to us wilful and cruel. Radiotherapy seemed the better option to us, and yet our opinion was not being considered and we had no direct contact with any radiologist in Brighton. [. . .]

Alex: I felt increasingly angry and hostile at this time, particularly towards Dr Cree, whom both Ann and I found immensely depressing to deal with – far more so than other doctors, who had been no more hopeful in their prognosis, but had approached our situation from a different perspective.

It was largely a problem of our simply not responding well to her personality, but sadly she was the only oncologist at the hospital and there was now no question of transferring Joe's care back to St Stephen's – he was no longer well enough to travel back and forth to London. As a result of this, the last months of Joe's life were more difficult for us to cope with than might otherwise have been the case. [. . .]

While Ann kept Joe occupied, I saw Dr Rodriguez alone in his office. We were desperate, and I know he sensed that, but I also felt that he was more sympathetic to our need to do something than Dr Cree was. I asked Dr Rodriguez a question which had scared the hell out of me whenever I thought about it: 'One of my biggest fears,' I said, 'is that the tumours on Joe's lungs will kill him, and that he'll die coughing up blood and be frightened. But what if the lung tumours don't kill him, what if somehow they stabilize and the tumours in his spine get worse? How can the bone tumours kill him? I can see how they can cause him immense pain – but how can they kill him?'

I sat watching Dr Rodriguez, partly because I thought I knew the answer. I knew the answer was horrible, but I wanted him to think about that horror – though it is only my presumption that he wasn't thinking about it anyway, since he knew far more than I ever would about the effects of cancer. I liked Dr Rodriguez and trusted him. He had young children himself, and both Ann and I felt more able to relate to doctors who were also parents; we felt that those parent–doctors showed a sympathy and an empathy that went beyond medical or even humanitarian concerns.

I hoped that facing up to this question, and the almost tangible gloom it seemed to throw over both of us in the room, might help persuade Dr Rodriguez to try anything, even a long shot, to help Joe.

Dr Rodriguez looked at me from behind his desk. 'The tumours might simply weaken Joe's spine to the point where it might snap, severing his spinal cord,' he said.

We stared at each other for a moment. This was a thought which had gone through my mind every time I had picked Joe up since his paralysis. I had a dread of actually causing him damage – or at the very least precipitating it. I tried to visualize what it might be like: me picking Joe up, his neck falling back or his spine collapsing beneath my grasp, Joe in an agony of pain, both of us terrified.

'Our main concern at the moment,' I said, 'is to find some way of reducing Joe's pain now. I think Ann and I know he's going to die, even if we block it all the time. But the drugs don't seem to work, and, in the short term, radiotherapy has helped him so much.'

Dr Rodriguez told me that there was one more possibility, a single session on something called a linear accelerator, which was more powerful than the normal radiotherapy equipment and which would irradiate the whole of Joe's thoracic region – below the neck and above the abdomen. One of the problems with Joe's continuing pain was that it was very difficult to isolate the source or sources. This high dose of radiation would hopefully hit the developing tumours wherever they were. It would mean that Joe's lungs would be irradiated, which could slightly impair his breathing, but this risk seemed outweighed by the possible benefits in terms of Joe's comfort. [. . .]

On Friday, 11 November, I took the train to London and went to Hammersmith and Queen Charlotte's. The entry in my diary for the day before records: 'Very negative day – exhausted, arguing with Ann.' This must have reflected the tension we were feeling, for we had very few rows during the course of Joe's illness.

Certainly, on the Friday, things seemed brighter. I met Mr Wood in his office at the hospital and explained, as thoroughly as I could, the stages of Joe's cancer. He, in turn, told me how he and his partners had developed Contracan as a result of research into the balance of saturated and unsaturated fat in the cells of cancer patients. He drew me a diagram and explained that this ratio had a direct bearing on cell death and the spread of cancer, and that clinical trials of Contracan to date had shown that it inhibited that spread, thus stabilizing the patient's condition.

He warned me that there was no evidence that it could do anything other than stabilize the cancer, but that several patients had reported greatly reduced pain and had been able to withdraw from morphine and other pain-killers. He emphasized again that he did not think Contracan could save Joe, but that it might help relieve his pain. Once Joe had had a 'base' X-ray from which his progress could be monitored, he was prepared to supply the suppositories, which we could administer ourselves at home, and there would be no charge for the treatment. He agreed that, if he were in my shoes, he would try anything that might help Joe, so long as it did not actually endanger him, and he felt that Contracan would not.

I had mentioned some of the difficulties we were having in dealing with Dr Cree, and Mr Wood stressed that I must talk to Ann and to Dr Cree before we went any further. Excited by even the remotest possibility that Contracan might help ease and prolong Joe's life – perhaps long enough that another treatment could be found – I called Ann from Queen Charlotte's and she agreed that I should call Dr Cree straight away.

I did so, from a pay phone in the Queen Charlotte's lobby, and was horrified by the total negativity of her response. She accused me of going behind her back, whereas before my meeting with Mr Wood I had known so little about Contracan that there would have been nothing to discuss. She said that she felt Mr Wood's behaviour – presumably, simply in meeting me – was unethical and made it clear that she felt any further trial for Joe was unwarranted and cruel. If we wanted to remove Joe from her care and place him under Mr Wood's (an impractical suggestion, as she well knew, given Joe's immobility now and our distance from London) then, fine, we could go ahead with Contracan, but she would not agree to it.

I asked her at least to think about the new treatment and to call Mr Wood, to which she responded that he could call her. I put the phone down, then immediately called Mr Wood and explained her reaction. He seemed unperturbed and was reassuring. He would talk to Dr Cree. I left the hospital and spent the afternoon in London in a foul temper, mentally cursing Dr Cree and feeling strongly that I would like to punch her.

My mood, certainly as far as Dr Cree was concerned, did not improve over the next few days, and was shared by Ann. We felt she had become a positive block to caring for Joe and we resented the fact that, whenever we talked to her, she sanctimoniously stressed that what was important was 'what's best for Joe', as if that was the furthest thing from our minds. No other doctor took this attitude, and we hoped that as parents we were sufficiently self-aware to weigh up our obvious, selfish wish that Joe should live and be with us, against the possibility that further treatment could actually impair the quality of what was left of his life.

[. . .]

When Dr Cree did call, I answered the phone. When she said she was thinking of coming round, I said 'No!' in no uncertain terms. I had never had the opportunity – or felt secure enough – to tell her a little of my feelings, but now seemed the time. I said that Ann and I were extremely angered by her reaction to the Contracan proposal, that we felt she was effectively exercising moral and emotional blackmail by suggesting that the only way we could proceed was by removing Joe from her care. I told her that we had grown increasingly unhappy about her attitude towards treating Joe, that we felt patronized by her, and that we were scared that her faith in God and Christian heaven meant that she was more willing to accept Joe's death than we were. 'We feel bludgeoned by your Christianity,' I said. I told her we had no faith in her any more and did not wish to deal with her or for Joe to see her.

I was so angry by the time I finished speaking to her that I was flushed and shaking. I felt slightly guilty at the hurt I must have caused her and knew that she was probably not as terrible as we thought, but at the same time, for whatever reasons, she had caused us immense, unnecessary pain and anxiety simply through her failure to respond to our needs as desperate parents. I went downstairs and told Ann about our conversation. Above all, we felt relieved that our feelings were out in the open and that we would no longer have to deal with Dr Cree.

THIRTY-NINE

'THE MEMORY BIRD': ACCOUNTS BY SURVIVORS OF SEXUAL ABUSE – EXTRACT 3

Anonymous (1) and Alex Benjamin (2)

1 EXTRACTS FROM A LETTER I SENT TO MY EX-THERAPIST

Dear Dr X

It is important to me that I let you know how I feel about my therapy with you, in the hope that I can finally put the experience behind me and move on.

I would like to ask you why you didn't believe me when I told you I was sexually abused as a child. I needed to explore my fears, but instead I felt alone. I was so confused that I even believed your version of reality, and felt that I must be very sick to 'imagine' that I was abused.

I needed someone to be there for me, to support me, and to accept what I was saying without getting angry and defensive. I didn't experience this acceptance with you. Instead, I felt as though I was wrong to tell you, that I was wasting your time as you weren't interested, and that I should just accept your terms, which was to avoid topics which you didn't want to talk about.

I have written to you in the hope that it will help me to be free of some of the destructive after-effects I have experienced from my experience of therapy with you. Although some of our sessions were helpful in terms of 'symptom management', on balance I think the negative effects have out-weighed anything positive I may have gained.

(Anonymous)

Source: Malone, C, Farthing, L, Marce, L. *The Memory Bird. Survivors of Sexual Abuse.* London: Virago Press, 1996. Reproduced by permission.

2 ABUSE: THE POWER OF ARTICULATING EXPERIENCES

Because doctor is always right and
we're crazy or mental cases or not
worth listening to and need drugs to
keep us quiet and if we say we've
been raped it's our own fault or we
made it up or we're having fantasies
and when we feel bad it's
part of our 'illness' not because we've
been abused and oppressed because
abuse doesn't exist and if they shout
at us or call us names it's 'therapy'
but if we feel angry or upset we're
being manipulative and because eventually
we may accept that they know best as what
choice do we really have and . . .
for lots and lots of other reasons it
is time to make them accountable and
acknowledge what they have done in
the name of therapy.

(Alex Benjamin)

FORTY

I DIDN'T KNOW HOW TO HELP HIM

Michele Hanson

When Nell Dunn's father was dying at home in great pain of a severe cancer, she found she was unable either to care for him physically or talk to him about what was going on. You would think that the author of *Up the Junction* and *Poor Cow* wouldn't have a problem with empathy and kindness, but Dunn feels that she has always been hopeless at it.

'My father didn't have a good death,' she says. 'I didn't know how to help him. I have never known how to support someone through a crisis and I wanted to be better at it, so I wrote the play *Cancer Tales* in order to learn how other people managed. I worked from the outset with director Trevor Walker, trying to create a dramatic form which authentically represented the lives of the people I had talked to.'

Cancer Tales is a series of monologues/dialogues – verbatim theatre, the voices of seven women and one man whose lives have been affected by cancer. Dunn calls them love stories, as they demonstrate what happens to relationships in the face of disaster. But with any life-threatening illness, not just cancer, your private life becomes public and you must also relate to doctors, nurses and many other members of the medical profession, some of whom may not be much good at relating either.

Dunn is fiercely opposed to 'doctor bashing'. 'We're expecting doctors to have a depth of kindness that I certainly haven't got,' she says. 'I'm impatient, irritable, forgetful, but they must be tremendously intelligent, generous and never forget anything. Some are not going to manage it. They are dealing, every day, with people who are depressed, ill, miserable, angry and frightened, and who need different things: "Tell me everything";

Source: *Guardian* 5 May 2003. Reproduced by permission.

"Don't tell me my son's going to die"; "Spend more time explaining"; "I don't want to talk to the doctor". Doctors have to feel their way. They make blunders because they're in the front line. We're hoping that doctors and nurses can be straightforward and kind all the time, but they can't. Why? Because they are often exhausted, working in a badly run system, overstretched, and to be generous every day is beyond human possibility.'

But is kindness something that can be taught? Actors are now being used in medical schools to role-play patients and then give medical students feedback. *Cancer Tales* has been performed for doctors, medical students and Macmillan nurses, and been very well received. It perhaps helps by illuminating the little things that make such a huge difference. 'I asked the anaesthetist: "Please will you whisper in my ear now and then that I'm doing very well",' says Clare, one of the characters in the play, 'and she said, "I will, even if they laugh at me." Also, when I was in the pre-op room, and they were putting needles in my veins, Mr Lawrence came out of the operating theatre wearing his funny little hat and said, "I want you to see. Look, I'm here." It says everything, doesn't it? He had a brusque manner . . . very gung-ho and matter of fact, yet he had that sensibility.'

Later, in a crowded radiotherapy waiting room, a young doctor must tell Clare about using a dilator to make her vagina stay open. She has never met this man before. 'I'm feeling absolutely shattered,' she says, 'I'm falling apart and trying not to show it, but I'm in a small space and all these people could hear everything. The women looked interested, the men hid their faces in their hands. I know the young doctor is doing his best in an impossibly undignified situation.'

'It's especially tough for the parents of grown-up children,' says Mary, whose daughter Rebecca is dying. 'You have a role but you can't really make any important decisions. It's very confusing how to be and where to be . . . I had to step back and not take control of her life. She wanted to be treated as a living person, not as a dying person.'

Dunn was in the position of a writer and outsider, but the people she was observing, stuck in the reality of serious illness, had to work it out for themselves, yet managed, somehow, in the most harrowing of situations, to be loving and generous. Joan had great difficulty looking after her adult son, who she could not believe was really ill. He kept hitting her – 'Not hard, just a sly punch' – and shouting at her. 'I was frightened to be alone with him, but he says, "Mum, you've got to give me a bath." I felt awful about that . . . I'd never seen him with no clothes on since he was little . . . anyway I help him, and I wash his back and he has a real nice bath . . . next day he wanted to go back to hospital and he never came out.'

When life really does become too short, you can't mess about any more, and every conversation takes on a heightened sensitivity. 'But our job is not to be overwhelmed by someone's misery,' says Dunn.

'We can acknowledge it, but still come in with good news about the outside world. If I went to the pictures last night and had a good time, I'm allowed to say so. Before I wrote this, I didn't know how to ask for support or how to give it,' she says. 'I'm managing better now, because I've learned how other people do it. Perhaps there isn't any extraordinary training – we just need to be straightforward and be ourselves. It's less exhausting.'

FORTY-ONE

SEPTEMBER 11TH: A PROFESSIONAL VICTIM

Anonymous

INTRODUCTION

September 11th is a date the world will not forget in a hurry: a date when potential air travellers will think twice about the necessity of their travel. September 11th 2001 was the date the Twin Towers which had dominated the New York skyline were destroyed, along with the innocent lives of the passengers on board the aircraft which crashed into those buildings, killing those who were in or around the two towering infernos at the time. It all happened in broad daylight. However, it was early night-time – what I call 'light darkness' – on September 11th five years earlier than the event I reflect on here occurred.

I had returned home after a formal conference dinner, connected with my academic role, having dropped off a colleague at her hotel. I had put my car in my garage and turned to close the garage door, when I realised that a youth was approaching me. He pointed out his accomplice, who was holding a gun. The first relieved me of my handbag. The second pushed me back into the garage and later persuaded the first youth to close the garage door after us. The latter having become very nervous, both at time passing and the apparent turn of events, ran off. My assailant, after pushing me into the back seat of my car, raped me at gun point. Horrific as this was, I managed to keep telling myself that I would survive and he was not going to kill me (it was only later that I thought of HIV). But the worst was yet to come. After getting out of the car, he could not open the garage door, and insisted I help him, pointing his gun at me, while I fumbled along the top of the door in the darkness. His panic was visibly mounting. I lost track of how long I was gripped by a rising fear that if I couldn't open the door to let him get out and away, or 'get through' to him, then the likelihood was that he would shoot both himself and me, as he threatened. Throughout the whole ordeal I kept talking to him, trying to calm him down, instinctively drawing on my long ingrained professional routine. I knew I had 'got through' to the first of my assailants. After all, he had contented himself with what I now imagine they had originally come for – the contents of my handbag. Needless to say, I did manage to open the door, more by fluke than design, and lived to tell the tale. It was only some time later that I discovered my attacker was profoundly deaf, having taken his hearing aid out to avoid easy identification. The fact that he was high on heroin was of little consequence in comparison to this barrier to communication. I knew I never reached him while I was his hostage.

All this had been five years earlier, but five years to the day. This was something that did not immediately occur to me until, in the immediate aftermath of the afternoon's shock waves, which had reverberated around our offices, I telephoned a close friend who worked for the Red Cross in London, partly to make reassuring contact, partly to check that London still existed, and for any information she might have. Her remark 'It's not a good date for you, is it?' was, I now realise, more pertinent and helpful than either of us would have imagined. She had made the connection that enabled me to anticipate that I might feel peculiarly and especially vulnerable, when I came down from my instinctive and automatic reliance on the professional role, which had carried me through the afternoon to that point. My social work training, from years before, had accustomed me to dealing with crises. While one of my colleagues went into immediate shock, and kept repeating 'It's World War Three!', I made the calming tea, and carried our joint supervision session with a student, which had gone ahead according to schedule.

My delayed and equally strong reactions might well have been overwhelming, but for my friend making the connection between the appalling carnage in the New World and my experience. The New York disaster involved thousands of people immediately, tens of thousands more through personal knowledge, a nation in shock and a world in recoil. My experience was small-scale, a life-threatening attack on an individual, me. While it only affected me immediately, some tens of people personally, and perhaps some more tens or hundreds who saw the local newspaper headlines, heard the local radio or saw the regional television news bulletins, the two incidents were inextricably linked in my experience. Obviously this was by date but, more importantly, by the shared experience of attack coming out of nowhere, being trapped and in mortal danger.

Any rekindling of such memories makes me permanently vulnerable to my subconscious mind going into what I now call 'shut down'. My mind goes into protective healing mode by cutting out all external and superfluous activity, what in lay language might be called shock or diagnosed by professionals as recurrent post-traumatic stress disorder. If I am able to predict or anticipate potential triggers then I can take appropriate measures and either ward it off or lessen its impact. But I first have to make a conscious connection between the wider experience and my own, in this instance September 11th 2001 in New York and September 11th 1996 in England.

That is precisely what my friend had enabled me to do. While I felt exceptionally vulnerable in the days following the destruction of the Twin Towers, I was able to take suitable preventive measures to avoid being incapacitated. In a sense I was lucky that time. My recall was confined to an intrusive memory, which I could understand if not control. Sometimes I've not had somebody to take such good care of me and failed to make the necessary connection myself. Full-blown flashbacks have set my anxiety soaring with attendant somatic disturbances. I've been unable to function normally, until I've understood the trigger and the aftermath subsided.

In the immediate aftermath six years ago, including the visit to the local police rape suite, I functioned almost on automatic professional pilot. The following morning I was able to ring my department and speak directly to one of the secretaries and explain why I would be unable to continue organising the conference. I then visited my GP. However, this ability did not last and I went into shock later in the day, and was less coherent with the two women CID officers who came to see me that afternoon than I had been with the uniformed officers the night before. Several days later, after giving my statement in many instalments, I went into a profound state of physical and psychological collapse. My muscles were either in spasm or failed to function properly. I had seized up physically. My stamina was zero. Most importantly of all, my thinking processes and concentration, normally sharp, were non-existent. I couldn't absorb or retain any new information, nor could I recall old and tried information, such as close friends' telephone numbers or even some names. Neither my short- nor my long-term memory was reliable. I've since likened the experience to a computer where the hard disk has been wiped. But, unlike a computer, where software can be reinstalled from CD-ROM, I had to be helped to reinstall my own programming and information, step by step, at my own pace, where I could feel safe and in control. It was painfully slow going. I was totally dependent for several weeks, unable even to plan and cook a meal. I started going into my workplace after four months, but did little other than shift a paper or two.

No sooner had I started to go into work than the police, who had been in continuous contact, rang to ask me to take part in an identity parade. They were pretty sure they had got my attacker. In the end he confessed, pleaded guilty and was sentenced the middle of the following year, and I was spared the possibility of having to give evidence. For the rest of the academic year I did no teaching, apart from the odd workshop. I very slowly finished off some research, did some marking and supervision and wondered if I could ever function as an academic again. The following academic year was spent testing that out. Returning from a trip abroad to visit relatives in April 1998, some 20 months after my September 11th, I decided 'recovery' was no longer an appropriate word to use. I could and had to function as I now was. There was no 'getting over it' or going back. I wasn't going to be able to work in the same way or at the same pace but I could work well enough.

Now I am writing six years on. Time enough for a necessary and substantial pause or what Williams (2002), in thinking about his experience of being a block away from the Twin Towers in New York on September 11th 2001, refers to as a 'breathing space', before reacting. For the first time I'm trying to think systematically and publicly about my experiences, reviewing the nature of helpful communications and relationships and those that were less helpful, seeing them in social context. This article draws on my personal September 11th experience outlined above, my professional social work training, several years of psychotherapy (started before 1996 in response to childhood issues, which had dogged me as an adult), and my expertise as an academic. My major professional aims have been, and continue to be, to understand social experience, especially that of people involved in health and community care services, and to encourage a range of human service professionals to develop a reflective, critical research-mindedness, appropriate to social context and with the aim of developing more responsive and appropriate services, both organisationally, collectively and at individual service user level. All through the lived experience of this episode I was trying to make intellectual sense, albeit in a rather disjointed, not very rigorous and haphazard way. It was what I did for a living and my personal therapy, started some time before, had encouraged me to try to understand my own inner reactions in relation to my historical, cultural and social environment. It was one way of trying to piece together my shattered sense of self: one I was only too accustomed to, even if not in quite such extreme circumstances.

In this article I am trying to practise what I have consistently preached. I am also experimenting by taking it a step further and reviewing my personal experience and inner world in the light of my professional self and external context. I draw on this experience to make some observations about the position of the professional, the impact of diversity and difference, and the importance of language and roles.

AN ATYPICAL VICTIM?

I think my experience of other professionals was atypical. My academic and employment status, my previous professional training and my general academic field were made immediately apparent to the police, as they started recording personal details. From the outset, I was a 'respectable and respected victim'. Unlike many rape victims, I never once felt that my word was being doubted, but I was relieved when the physical examination proved the reality of what had happened.

The attitude of the police who attended immediately was exemplary and the uniformed women police constables who stayed with me until I returned home several hours later, after being taken to the 'rape suite' for examination and to make an initial statement, were outstanding. Later on, I even wrote to the chief constable to say so. For example, I was able to take the initiative and say that I did not wish to see a particular police surgeon, not because I doubted his professional capacity, but because he was known to me personally. The police even drove me around while he was sent away, to ensure there was no chance we should encounter each other. I wondered how many other rape victims have been able to claim personal knowledge of the police surgeon? However, I had not been offered any choice. It was pure chance that, as we arrived at the rape suite, one of the officers remarked, on seeing a male figure in the distance, 'Oh, there's the police surgeon. He's here already.' I thought he looked familiar and, on asking his name, my suspicions were confirmed.

During the whole episode I was always able to respond to the police officers, of whatever rank, doctors, nurses, victim support staff, my psychotherapist, the insurance broker, the loss adjuster and probation officers as fellow professionals. Once I had come off my automatic pilot stance of the first few hours, it seemed as though I could always access my sense of professional worth and esteem, despite being only too aware that my body and mind had collapsed round me. I could say what I wanted. I knew I needed help. I expected the best from the professionals and probably got it.

The police were constantly in my life. I wondered whether I was a 'preferential victim'. They took great pains to keep me in contact with the case. However, as with all police officers, they tended to call round when it suited them, without contacting me first to check whether it was convenient. This might be appropriate with suspects, but it is not always with victims. In the event, I got used to our Saturday evening cups of coffee and sort of enjoyed them.

While my specific academic area is not criminology, I knew enough of how to work professionally with a range of health and welfare professionals. I had the 'know how'. I knew if what they were doing made sense and if it seemed appropriate. Furthermore, I had access to colleagues who did know about the criminal justice system. When the police were unable to get information about the progress of the case, especially when sentencing was likely, my contacts were able to access it, enabling me to inform the police. If there was anything I needed by way of contacts or information, I was often in a position to obtain it. For example, a friend worked at the local sexually transmitted diseases clinic. A few days after my attack, she arranged for a female consultant she respected and rated very highly to check me over and carry out the required HIV test. My friend, a nurse, offered to come into the examination room with me but, while on most occasions welcoming the support of the female friends who accompanied me to all such significant encounters, in this instance I decided on a little more professional distance. Later and in other situations I was less concerned. Under the Criminal Justice and Disorder Act 1998, the Probation Service are required to contact victims of serious crimes. The officer assigned to me was a friend of a friend. If we met socially, which we did very occasionally, I used to delight in referring to 'my probation officer'.

Most importantly of all, I also had access to a therapist I knew and trusted and who knew my background. I cannot imagine how important, but demanding, it must be to start a counselling relationship at the same time as dealing with the immediate aftermath of such an experience. In summary, I had enormous professional resources at my disposal.

Significantly, I had sufficient material resources to be able to afford extra help at the time when I needed it. My job was safeguarded and my salary still came when I was off sick. I could afford to buy a new car, even before the insurance money came. While I eventually received criminal compensation, it came too late to be used to pay for the immediate therapeutic help I had needed and did not cover my costs. I was, of course, out of pocket, but I considered it money well spent.

DIVERSITY AND DIFFERENCE

I am a middle-aged white woman who was attacked by a young black man. Professionally I was only too aware of the over-representation of young men from minority ethnic groups in our prisons, mental hospitals and among those apprehended by the police. I can remember saying to one of the first neighbours to help me, 'They would have been black, wouldn't they?' My response later was to become even more angry than I already was at the outrage, when I thought that I had tried to be aware of ethnic issues in my work. They had chosen one of the wrong kind!

It did not help that the police surgeon who saw me immediately after was not only a man but also Asian. He was very calm and kind, and only too aware that a female doctor would have been more appropriate. Apparently there were no female police surgeons working for that particular police authority. I was never more grateful for sustained, gentle, careful but disciplined female presence than that provided by the two uniformed policewomen who stayed with me as I went through the tortuous procedures that all rape victims go through, as all evidence is carefully gathered. They then took me to where I was staying in the middle of the following night. The next day two women CID officers interviewed me at length and took over police contact with me. Giving the detailed statement that was required in the days following was difficult enough, but it would have been made doubly difficult if I had been required to work with a male police officer, however sensitive. Some months into the case the senior female officer on my case was moved to another station. There being no available female officer to replace her, a male officer was assigned to work with me. This was handled with tact. I was warned and apologies were offered. By this stage I thought it would probably be helpful to work with a male officer. Since the attack, I had been having intensive therapy with the male therapist I had already been working with before the attack. I had been able to keep male–female contact going and had consciously retreated from any help that might have affected cross-gender communication. In the event, the male police officer proved to be the most sensitive of all the police in realising my perspective and what information I needed from him to progress my life: often little things, for example how could I retrieve things like maps and my road atlas, which had been in my car, or when could my insurance company get to view my car (subsequently it was a write-off after the forensic services had torn it apart). It was him who arranged for the crime prevention officer to visit at my request.

Immediately after the attack, the police asked me to categorise whether my attacker was African–Caribbean or Asian. I got it wrong. I did develop a pretty accurate photo-fit likeness, though, with the aid of a police computer program the following week. I couldn't help thinking what a useless way to characterise an individual. I had been sitting next to some people from the Middle East at the dinner earlier that evening of September 11th. How do you categorise them? African or Asian? What about people of mixed race?

Even now I find myself being wary of young black men in the street, especially at night. My reactions more immediately after the incident, while being understandable, bordered on the completely racist. I was appalled when collecting a colleague's children from their nursery class to encounter a playground populated by many young black boys. As my panic rose, I immediately assumed it was a breeding ground for little rapists! Sustained exposure to this situation did desensitise me, but I avoided any situation at work that might result in me being alone in my office with a black male student for a considerable time.

I was fortunate in finding a female black massage therapist to work with me pretty soon after the attack. Once the initial shock had subsided, I could hardly move and felt totally dissociated from my body. I knew people who did massage and I already had a psychotherapist in whom I had total confidence. I was, however, convinced that I needed somebody who could cope with me shaking and trembling as I still frequently did, and who could cope with my mind–body trauma. My networks, previously mentioned, provided a name. I telephoned and made an appointment. It was only when I arrived that I realised she was black. Given the state I was in at the time, I doubt if I would have gone if I had known in advance. In fact it has proved to be one of the most healing encounters of my life and I still go for massage.

Reflecting back on all these experiences now, I am more than aware that the stereotypical and racist reactions I felt and voiced in the heat of the moment of the attack, and which appalled me, even at the time, were the product of intense fear and terror. At the same time as experiencing them, I knew they were irrational, but I was incapable of engaging my usual rational and indeed experientially grounded understanding and expectations of good interactions with black and minority ethnic people. These had formed part of my daily life for a very long time.

SHARING THE LANGUAGE

I have already described how 'professional speak' was familiar to me. I understood the terms and the jargon of some professional organisations and systems. Over the months, I learned a lot about the life of the police, probably more than they learned about the academy. I completely failed to enable them to understand the nature of research evidence. When some DNA results came back, they read me parts of the report, complaining about the scientifically accurate and necessarily cautious interpretation of the results. They wanted definitive evidence – 100% certainty, not 'probably', 'likely' or 'on the other hand'. They were action people. What they called paperwork, which always forms a large part of my daily work, was of much lower priority and of little interest. While I am by nature a reflective thinker, using theoretical understanding pragmatically, they wanted direct activity. I suppose between us, if we could have joined forces we would have made a good team, in that teams are ideally supposed to consist of a variety of types of people.

Sometimes there was no adequate language. There was no way people could express the impact of the seriousness of their concern. Words seemed limp. Friends and family could use touch but professionals could not. Several police officers commented that it was one of the worst rape scenarios they had dealt with. I learned of their concern and involvement by implication. At such times I found myself needing to translate into emotional terms the implications of their individual rational comments. After my attacker had been arrested, one woman police officer confessed to being a bit verbally 'rough' with him, and that she had felt like 'throttling him'. I had got to know this officer pretty well by this time. I also needed to translate the language of systems at a symbolic level. I interpreted the severity of his sentence as an important indication of the seriousness of what had happened to me. While I doubted the therapeutic effect of a

long-term prison sentence, and knew the way sex offenders were frequently treated by other inmates often made it necessary for them to be in
isolation, which in itself was only likely to brutalise, I needed to accept the
language of the criminal justice system on its own terms and within its
own frame of reference. This was the only way it could acknowledge me. I
might have wished that society took my situation seriously according to
my understanding of the social factors behind offending and that sex
offenders, while clearly needing containment, also desperately need deep
rehabilitation and help. Similarly, the judge's summing-up speech was a
public recognition of my trauma.

At times, I think, my professional standing and apparent articulate
ability was a barrier to communication, especially with the police. I was
still a victim of a very serious crime with all the physical, and emotional
turmoil that entailed. A cognitive response was probably easier for them
than a felt or an emotional response. I remember in the early weeks, as I
was being driven by one of the women police officers, she started a conversation. Without thinking, she asked me whether I had yet been into work.
I couldn't believe my ears. I was barely functioning in any respect. Not
normally a nervous passenger or driver, I was already finding her steady
30 mph faster than I could cope with and feeling giddy. I replied, somewhat testily, 'I work with my head. I can't watch the shortest television
programme or read even a few sentences of a newspaper.' She never asked
again. It was, I suspect, a classic case of knowing intellectually about the
psychological effects of rape and trauma but 'selectively forgetting' in the
situation. At later times I was to be shocked occasionally by colleagues,
many of whom know a great deal about mental health issues, apparently
divorcing their academic and intellectual knowledge from their lived
reality as they encountered me back in the workplace. In part, this was a
measure of the institutional pressure on them to 'just get on with the job',
which of course it was for me too, or rather in the early stages to test out
whether I could. These days I know I can, but I still have to live with the
unpredictable effects.

In the early days, though, I did wonder about the police, who were the
professionals I was most in contact with, perhaps being deceived by my
apparent capability and ability to discuss my situation. Similarly, those
close to me were also traumatised. While we could appear rational and
receptive to instructions, I would immediately forget what I had been
told and agreed to. My carers were equally prone to 'mis-hear'. Leaflets
about victim support services, rape crisis counselling services, and police
services were very useful, but more written information specific to our
circumstances, for example when the police wanted to interview me
again or when more information was to be released to the media, would
have been very useful. I would argue for all kinds of duplicate and overlapping communications to be used with trauma victims and those near
them.

One of the most useful things was being able to piece together the story of what happened. When I was told that giving my initial statement could take up to about 20 hours I could not credit it. Many exhausting hours later I had a clearer picture of the narrative. It was not yet 'my' story. The expression and grammar would not have been of my choosing, but it proved to be a first step, the first of many. This article now is another. Similarly, putting together a pre-sentencing statement of the impact of the crime on my functioning and abilities enabled me to tell my story and summarise its effects.

With friends and especially in therapy I was able to develop a much fuller story, piecing together an emotionally valid and intellectually coherent understanding of the impact of this story within the story and context of my life. Fortunately, I was accustomed to talking about my emotions, but some of those around me were less so. I mentioned above that some academic colleagues appeared to dissociate their intellectual knowledge from their encounters with me. I remember being at work, when the police rang to tell me they had arrested a suspect and could I do an identity parade the following day. I made a chance remark to a male colleague that I could kill my attacker. Much to my surprise this mild man responded ferociously that he could do so as well. Remembering how female colleagues had described the reactions of some of my male colleagues, I found myself recognising that if my attacker had been placed in a room with these intellectually sophisticated and normally gentle men, he might not have survived. It gave me new insight into the genesis of lynch mob violence. At a later date, I certainly found thumping my massage therapist with a pillow, while pretending that she was my attacker, very cathartic, demonstrating the need to understand and communicate about such a life-threatening and changing experience, verbally and non-verbally, intellectually and emotionally.

A MATRIX OF ROLES

There were times when I felt as if I was at the centre of a complicated socio-gram of professional contacts, or the centre of a pie chart, whose segments did not quite meet either in the centre or along their sides. There were gaps, and in the gaps there was my life.

It took me a while to realise that each professional group had their own task, their own agenda, which, while important, was not necessarily mine. For example, the police, who were the group I had most contact with in the early days, were always very concerned about my welfare, even giving me their mobile phone numbers and instructing me to feel free to call night or day. But, as I took more and more charge of my life I slowly recognised what is after all obvious, but not to me initially, that their primary task was to apprehend my attacker, whereas mine was to rebuild my confidence, stamina and mental wellbeing. Sometimes to do that I needed practical information from them, which was a while coming, because although it was important to my task it was not to theirs. Of all the professionals involved in my recovery it was my therapist who held the pieces of the pie chart together and saw the importance of the whole.

The concept of a professional who is also a victim was complicated. At times it seemed that other professionals had difficulty holding my two roles in mind simultaneously. When I was being the victim, I needed help and support, but when I began to reflect on or analyse my situation, which was a very natural tool for me to use in making sense of my experience, and as a way of aiding my recovery, then it was harder for health and welfare professionals, who had only known me in this context, to remember I was also a victim.

This led me to think about the need for ongoing support for those professionals working with service users who had been exposed to trauma. There were a couple of weeks when neither policewoman contacted me, despite having promised to do so. When one eventually telephoned to apologise and reeled off a list of the horrific crimes she had been dealing with in the intervening time, I wondered what support they had. I know they had said my case was one of the worst of its kind they had to deal with, and I guess they identified with me as a victim, perhaps because I was a fellow human service professional, more than they did with many other victims they encountered. However, any empathy offered to victims is inevitably going to affect their inner worlds too.

Professional relationships have boundaries that personal ones do not have. When my attacker was sentenced, the police officers assigned to my case were in court. They came to see me afterwards to share their reactions. Even the female police officer who had been moved to another station rang me. The sentence, although severe, was in their collective opinion justified. They were very satisfied. It signified a job well done. I can't remember whether they had a drink that day. I would have offered it. They may have still been on duty. But their intention was clear. This was cause for celebration. However, we had lost the reason for our contact. These officers had been my constant companions for months. I had grown accustomed to our coffee sessions. We all knew that, although there would be minor formalities to complete, it was time to separate, but lingered over doing so. As they left, for the first time ever I walked to the police car and waved them off.

One role I would not have anticipated was that of being a teacher. Medical and nursing staff at my local GP surgery, responsible for my continued medication and tests, and personnel staff at my place of work have commented that they learned much of what they know about the impact of trauma, from what I have been able to tell them. I hope this article might have a similar use.

CONCLUSION

The work of all the professionals within my 'helping' constellation was important. However, the consistent, continuous, 'for as long as it takes', 'at my pace', dependable and intelligent help from my therapist was fundamental, neither minimising the horror nor wallowing in it, but providing a quiet and steadfast belief in the future, my future – not a perfect future but one that could encompass the positive, the negative and the neutral tones, that need to go together. It certainly provided us with at least a two-year or longer detour in our journey, which we would not have anticipated, and which took us to places we would not otherwise have gone.

As for me, I now see myself in professional terms as able to function, not at the same pace or level as before, but I'm not a weak link. Certainly, I'm vulnerable when I least expect it but, if the worst hits me, once I can understand the trigger, and take the necessary steps and time, I know I'm on my way back. My colleagues are beginning to know this too. But, like dog ownership, this sort of experience is for life. There is no going back. This is my life.

REFERENCE

Williams, R. (2002) *Writing in the Dust: Reflections on 11th September and Its Aftermath*, London, Hodder and Stoughton.

FORTY-TWO

REPRODUCING SUBJECTIVITY AND MEANING IN NURSING WORK

Jane Seymour

Mr Albert Randall had been admitted to the intensive care unit at Western Hospital following surgery for a perforated duodenal ulcer. ... Here we [join] the situation the day after it had been decided by medical staff that 'active treatment' would no longer be given. It is the general shift handover from the night staff to the 'early' staff. The charge-nurse, Z, who has been caring for Mr Randall overnight, is speaking:

Z: 'We've turned him about three times, his feed is still going and he's on ten breaths [of the ventilator]. I didn't adjust the ventilator down any more, because I think he would go quickly, and I didn't think it was fair to telephone his wife at 3 or 4 o'clock in the morning.'

At the bedside Z hands over in more detail to Nurse A and they talk about how best to manage his death:

A: 'What do you think I should do Z? Should I, am I allowed to take his et. [endo-tracheal] tube out?'
Z: 'No you can't, but boy, did I want to. I think it looks gross ... I really wish we could get it out and make him look really nice for his wife. We can't take it out without the doctors' say so though.'
A: 'What about telephoning his wife, when should I do that?'
Z: 'Well, if I were you, I'd wait until about 09:00 and then put him on a "t" piece, turn off the pressure support [accepted techniques of

Source: Seymour, JE. *Critical Moments: Death and dying in intensive care.*
Buckingham: Open University Press, 2001.

reducing respiratory support in what is known as a "terminal wean" situation], and then call his wife – it won't be long then.'

(From the field notes)

Nurse A is left at this point to try to carry through these plans. The following section examines the way in which she attempted to do this, while simultaneously being required to carry out the more medically led plans for Mr Randall, focusing particularly on the account she gave of the events in her follow-up interview.

After the charge-nurse Z leaves, Nurse A is left alone to look after Mr Randall. She speaks to another nurse and to myself (I have been listening to the bedside handover) about her plans: she says that she has decided to wait until Mrs Randall phones the unit, rather than telephoning Mrs Randall herself. She voices the hope that he will stay 'stable' in the meantime, and says that she will not put him on a 't" piece until she hears that Mrs Randall is on her way to the hospital. She makes ready to wash Mr Randall, drawing the curtains around the bed:

A: 'I'm going to make a start and get him washed and looking good, so that when she does ring, we're all ready.'

(From the field notes, day 10)

Having drawn these plans, events do not unfold in the way that A expects, and she becomes increasingly anxious. Mrs Randall does not telephone the unit as A hopes. Then she is asked by the medical staff to remove the ventilator from Mr Randall. A attempts to contact Mrs Randall before she takes the ventilator away, and gets no reply to her call. She eventually takes Mr Randall off the ventilator at 11:30, without his wife being present. She carefully ensures that he is breathing comfortably without the ventilator, adjusting the tubing attached to his endo-tracheal tube to ensure that there is no obstruction to the flow of air. I realize that she is upset and decide to leave in order to avoid adding to her stress.

When the ventilator has been removed, A carefully checks Mr Randall to make sure he is comfortable. He flickers his eyes and moves slightly and she talks reassuringly to him. She starts to write her report, head bent and avoiding eye contact with anyone. Other nurses keep coming and asking her to keep an 'eye' on their patients (who are deemed more in need of attention because they are more 'sick'?) while they get drugs or have a break. I go over to tell her that I will leave after the pm handover and wait while she finishes writing. I start to speak and then realize that she is very, very distressed. I ask her if she is OK and she starts to cry – I put my arm around her, and she tells me that she is feeling very unhappy:

> *I can't get hold of his wife and I really think that he might die without her being here. I think she ought to have the opportunity to*

*come in. Now I've been told to take him off the vent, and I really feel
like I am killing him – I think it's partly because I looked after him the
other day and I felt he was responding a bit to me, and even now, he's
flinching at times –' She cries more.*

I try to reassure her, that she has tried her best to contact Mrs Randall and
how comfortable he looks. I apologize that I cannot do anything to help
her sort the situation out but advise her that she needs to talk to the nurse
in charge. She is reluctant to do this, but allows me to speak to the 'f'
grade staff nurse. I do this as tactfully as I can, and then return with some
tissues for her. She is calmer now, and I get my bag ready to leave.

As I am leaving. I see the 'f' grade taking A into the 'quiet' room, she
nods at me. A is crying again.

(From the field notes, day 10)

One month after these events I am able to interview A about her recollections. She gives an account of why the situation was so difficult for her,
explaining it in terms of her intimate 'knowledge' about Mr Randall
'himself', her desire to achieve the 'right' kind of death for him, and her
lack of understanding about, and control of, the process of decision
making surrounding his death. She starts her account by explaining how
'depressed' she was that Mr Randall had been transferred eventually to a
ward (rather than dying on intensive care):

A: *'The thing that really got me lately was Mr Randall; you know about
    him anyway. The thing that really got me there was at the end of the
    shift they transferred him to the ward and – I don't know – that was
    the hardest thing I've had to deal with on here because it was depress-
    ing. I didn't feel like I was getting anywhere, it was just depressing.'*
JS: *'Can you tell me what it was like for you when you were involved in
    his care?'*
A: *'Well, I'd actually looked after him the previous week on nights and
    came back onto days and looked after him again. That was my choice.
    I wanted to do it because I felt like he knew me; because now and
    again he would open his eyes, and I just wanted to be there for him. I
    wanted him to know that I was there. I think also, that dying patients,
    some nurses don't let them know that they are there, just by, you
    know, touch, holding his hand, stuff like this, and I wanted to do that,
    just so as he knew that he wasn't on his own. His wife didn't want to
    be there – although I didn't know that until the day I thought he was
    actually going to die. So I don't know, I felt like the pressure was on
    me. His wife didn't want to be there, I'd tried to contact her, I'd said
    to her the previous night: 'If you go out tomorrow, leave me a*

number' and she didn't. So it was obvious that she didn't want to come in. I just felt like I was – I don't know – the only person he'd got. Do you know what I mean? To sort of see him out ... and he reminded me of my granddad [slight embarrassed laugh] as well. And the fact he was an alcoholic. When I'd looked after him on nights, someone said, "Oh, yeah, he's an alcoholic, and he's needed heminevrin down on the ward", and that sort of blackens your view; and yet, when it came to it and I'd spoken to his wife, it turns out that he wasn't like that at all; he might have been like it in hospital when he was ill, but at home he used to go down and help these homeless people who were alcoholic as well. You know, he did a lot of good work. I thought, bloody hell, I've thought badly of you, and I should- n't have done at all ... I just felt so sorry for him, he looked so child- ish lying there and he had his eyes open now and again, and I thought, "Christ, I ought to be telling him he's dying, does he know?" In case there was anything he wanted to say – he probably couldn't speak, but maybe mouth something ... they'd already withdrawn when I came on duty that day, but what got me was that he was a bit more with it and I just thought, are they doing the right thing?'

(From follow-up interview)

A's ideal of death is revealed here – physical contact with a close, 'known' individual, facilitation of communication, knowledge of imminent dying. She interprets Mrs Randall's absence in a particular way, feeling that the burden to achieve this sort of death then falls on her shoulders alone. Her memory of her grandfather further forges a sense of connection with Mr Randall and imbues her relationship with him with a sense of intimacy, so much so that she requests to be allowed to care for him. This ideal death, for her, must also be intelligible according to, as she sees it, her 'basic' understanding of medicine, and yet this is not so: she remembers not understanding why the withdrawal of treatment is being carried out, and not being provided with the explanations that she needs to make sense of events:

A: *'Er, the thing is, because you think, feel, that the doctors know every- thing, I'd said to them, look, well, he's more, well, he seemed more with it neurologically, and even one of the doctors thought that as well. I think he had second thoughts about withdrawing, and you think Christ, if he [the doctor] is, why don't they try and start to treat him again ... if a doctor thinks that he might make it, then, you know. But they still didn't ... maybe they could have explained things a bit better to people like me, I mean I've got a basic understanding, so if they'd explained it better then maybe I could've coped with it better myself, you know.'*

(From follow-up interview)

Thus for A, her work with Mr Randall becomes a source of stressful contradiction: her ideal of what constitutes nursing care for a dying person means that she sets the task for herself of 'being there for him' as he dies. She indeed achieves a particular sense of closeness to him, imagining that he is a 'known' person, much like her own, loved grandfather. She takes on the burden of trying to engender a situation where his wife is 'with him' and close to him, and finds it incomprehensible when Mrs Randall does not respond in the way she expects. When she has to carry out what to her is the final, illogical withdrawal of technological support; all of the intimacy that she has crafted so carefully is compromised. She recalls that: *'I suppose I felt like I was killing him'*, and, with his transfer out of intensive care to be nursed by strangers, the connection is finally broken between herself and Mr Randall.

This situation involved the struggles of a relatively inexperienced nurse who was attempting to deliver 'nursing' to a man from whom medical attention had been withdrawn formally. [. . .]

FORTY-THREE

TEXT APPEAL

Charis Alland

To be suddenly struck by a poverty of speech is, to someone whose life has evolved around conversation, to be plunged into deep water when you're unable to swim – the sense of drowning, the loss of solid ground, terrifying. The only noise is the babble of water spluttering over you as you sink deeper and deeper beyond a place where sound has meaning.

I would have considered finding myself in such a place the nightmare I never dared imagine. Yet find myself there I did. A place where sound merely echoed the hollow empty void of life as I perceived it – nothing but an illusion of connection in an alien, dissociated space. Out of depth and lost from sight, without a voice, in a tumultuous sea, a message in a bottle is, perhaps, the only hope. The challenge is to find the bottle that successfully transports the signal home.

Speech is so fundamental to our lives. As a therapist, language had been my everyday tool that empowered; as a sufferer from depression, it became the fool's gold – limiting and worthless. Locked in a world, silent of hope, I felt lost and bereft of the medium for expression that we depend on for conveying to each other the essence of our lives – linking us to humanity. Inventing a different point of departure, away from the demands of talking, which would reach out and be understood, required a creative energy that was hard to find.

In the confines of a mental hospital I withdrew. For three months I was on constant observation – a nurse at my side 24 hours a day. The will to find a bottle and define a message was difficult. My only communication with the outside was via the ward telephone (when it worked) or my mobile phone. It was the latter that soon became my unexpected lifeline – offering me the vehicle for maintaining contact with my previous existence. Without it my former life may have disappeared beyond recognition.

For a while I limited contact with friends and family. Face-to-face my well-developed mask was a master in the art of deception. I could smile and nod, hug and laugh, gesticulate and intonate – just as I always had. Hiding behind habitual social responses I found it impossible to admit to the depths of despair and felt an obligation to act on urges to reassure and protect others from my problems. My inner life was in conflict with the one others witnessed. In hospital I was freed from the pressure and stripped bare of the suprasegmental and paralinguistic language that, far from giving me away, was my cover. In this new space I was removed from the comfortable and familiar ways of relating to others. It provided the challenge to take more risks, experiment and be more honest with myself.

So why text?

It was, maybe, what most would consider the biggest limitation of text that held the greatest appeal for me. The need to be concise and economical with words helped in my bid to avoid expansion or explanation and yet made it possible to keep in contact. This was an advantage not afforded by telephone or face-to-face contact, where silences hung heavily, their meaning often interpreted erroneously. Brevity was also less difficult to defend in the case of email or snail mail – perhaps the exception being a postcard! Depending on others for access to stationery or the internet didn't make these favourable options. Sending a text was half the price of a stamp and, with little to say and no income, an important consideration. Poor concentration also made text the option of choice.

As I became unwell the disparity between my outer and inner life grew. Unwittingly my words had followed the unconscious deception of my voice and body. I had always placed a high value on integrity and believed that this lay, ultimately, in being truthful in what I said. Little did I understand how my use of words had been so influenced by a hidden emotional landscape. Focusing on a minimal use of words I realised how much I had avoided voicing my own thoughts in favour of saying what I thought others wanted to hear. Once in hospital the necessity of protecting myself from responding to other people's needs played a large part in appreciating this distinction.

In the beginning my exchanges were very brief, mostly apologetic, anxious not to reject or abandon people or lose my defining role as carer of their needs:

'Sory cant come 2 fone but ok hope u r feeling beta'; 'not up 2 tlking but gd 2 b in contact'; '0thing personal but 2 tired 2 tlk'; 'plse keep in contact'; 'how r u/yr family/hols/course'; 'sory to let u down will fone wen I can'.

Slowly I learned, from the various responses, to differentiate between those people I could open up to and depend on a little more, and those I needed to hold in a 'waiting space' until I had regained the strength and energy to respond on the more equal or lighter footing the friendship required. Understanding that we form various kinds of relationships, all of which can occupy some place in our lives, was important for me.

With some friends and family I could deflect the attention away from myself very easily and be distracted by their lives. Responses to my texts were based on giving me news of their lives:

> *'going on hol 2moro'; 'son past his xams'; 'horid day at wrk'; 'have flu'; 'moving hse'; 'granddaughter born today!'*

With others I was encouraged (and sometimes positively pushed!) to reach out and ask for help and be supported by them:

> *'never mind me how r u'; 'u v hlpd me now my turn to support u'; 'hold on life can b gd'; 'I want 2 hlp'; 'don't 4get u r a special person 2 me'; 'u have come so far don't give up now'.*

These were perhaps the scariest and most challenging for me! Gradually (and suspiciously) I began to reach out to those people, eventually asking more openly for help. My texts evolved from 'don't want 2 burden u', 'u have enuf on yr plate' to

> *'wd like 2 tlk'; 'plse fone'; 'in state can u fone'; 'want 2 leave here now'; 'wld like 2 c u'; 'HELP!'*

There were, of course, some who fell in between the two and I began to recognise how other people protected themselves when they needed space. So I came to understand, and not be offended or rejected, when even those who most wanted to help needed to hold back and could not respond:

> *'unable to fone u 2nite need space but stil care'; 'bad day 4 me but wil keep in touch'; 'u r worthy of time and love but I can't c u this w/e'.*

It gave me permission to feel less guilt when I needed to do the same with others. Text played a vital role in this – it allowed both distance and intimacy, giving other people, as well as me, space to decide how to respond.

Without punctuation or room to expand, text messages can often be ambiguous. Sometimes this leads to confusion and misunderstandings but there are also advantages. Sometimes I felt ambivalent, unsure of what I needed or why I wasn't able to talk to or see people. 'Unable 2 come 2 fone' offered little by way of a reason. It may have been that I was too physically tired or ill; that I was expecting to meet someone; that the phone was out of order; that I didn't want to speak; that I didn't want to talk in front of the particular person who was observing me; or a combination of all these and more! Conveying the message without having to explain was a relief and helped assuage the guilt I automatically felt when I rejected people. It was unusual for them to interrogate further. Strangely a message was accepted without the questioning that quite often accompanied a similar exchange by telephone. Those who did ask were usually just needing reassurance that I was OK and not becoming more unwell. I was able to create space without guilt and gain some privacy.

Privacy in a state psychiatric hospital, particularly when under 24-hour observation, is a concept that is almost extinct! Even without the observations, there is often not the physical space to have a confidential conversation with family or friends. Until the Care Standards fully come into their own, bed space is usually in dormitories and out of bounds to visitors; public telephones are situated in corridors; and communal rooms, by the very nature of being in an acute ward in a mental hospital, tend to be noisy, disruptive places. When I worked in psychiatry I often wondered how it was that some survivors of the system could be so non-discerning about disclosing personal details of their life to anyone in any situation. It is, perhaps, because it becomes the norm to talk in public places about deeply personal issues. I would be asked intimate questions in corridors, at the dinner table or when in the television lounge. I found it deeply invasive and offensive but seldom made any objection. Text gave me some feeling of privacy and control as well as an illusion of space. It helped me learn that I could create personal space in the most challenging and claustrophobic circumstances; it endorsed and protected my right to choose with whom I shared certain information.

Talking to family and friends retrospectively, I discovered how useful a medium it had been for them too. Some found the concept of mental illness difficult to handle and I may have lost contact with them if we had relied on visits or phone calls. Text was less threatening to those people, providing some distance and allowing them to dictate the terms of their contact with me. They were able to respond in a way they could handle and in their own time (and vice versa). A letter provides a similar facility but we seldom have the space needed for writing and posting a letter these days.

For some of these people I realised that it, incidentally, challenged their preconceptions about mental illness. Being able to recognise (from my texts) the me they knew so well, while at the same time acknowledging what was going on for me, enabled them (and me) to realise I had not become an alien! Others would ignore my illness and continue to relate to me as if there was nothing wrong. I learned to accept this, valuing enough the kind of relationship we had not to challenge or personalise their responses, but I did limit my replies to times when I felt stronger.

For those I grew to trust with more of the internal torment of my world, it was a useful way for them to support me and at the same time protect themselves – particularly when they had little energy for the strain that undoubtedly went with conversations when I was at my bleakest. In turn, I respected the distance they needed.

Through the use of text my relationships evolved and grew immensely. I learned to trust people in different ways, not make assumptions, and accept more readily the care, support and intimacy offered. Respecting the different ways people responded helped me discover and appreciate the unique and individual contributions they made to my life.

There were, of course, lots of problems. Not least was the challenge of needing my mobile recharged; it would disappear into a plethora of mobiles in the nursing office – sometimes to be lost for days! To begin with I was living in the fantasy world of instantaneous transmission. So when I asked for someone to call and received no reply I would be cata-strophically catapulted into abandonment and rejection. Text delay was something I had to learn to live with. It enabled me to challenge my predilection for jumping to conclusions. Lack of punctuation, irregular spelling and shorthand were other confusional delights! Texts such as 'looking 4ward 2 c-ing u sat gd' would leave me wondering whether it referred to the person seeing me on Saturday or that the previous Saturday had been good. Sometimes I'd send a text and receive a 'yes' response several days later, having forgotten the original question!

And then there were the technophobes! Among them were those unable to turn off the predictive text; those who I am sure thought text would bite if they wrote more than one word; and those who feared that putting their name to a text might incriminate them in some way! It led to some amusing guessing games and detective work.

As someone who had loved words, I gradually began to regain my fasci-nation with language. The irregular spelling reminded me of the English of Chaucer's era. I have often been amazed we have persevered so long, in our world of convenience, with spelling that contains complicated rules and is not phonetic. Could it be that we are now on the edge of a long-awaited textual revolution?

I had always detested mobile phones. I once thought of them as the most loathsome form of communication. I hated them for their intrusive-ness; for contributing to a feeling that we have to be constantly available; for the noise pollution and possible health risks. In a way, developing a different kind of relationship with them mirrored my own development – providing an analogy to the progress I made in therapy. I learned to seek out the supportive and nourishing things in the midst of hopelessness – holding out for the lifeboat in stormy waters. Appreciating that not everything is black or white, good or bad, opened me to the full spectrum of life and relationships – not just the extremes. Through text I saw the positives in something I had so loathed and through my journeying I began to see the possibility of liking the person I had so nearly destroyed.

FORTY-FOUR

GOING THE EXTRA MILE

Nicki Cornwell

I'm an interpreter. I work for a local authority, and am booked by health and local authority workers for interviews with users of their services who have little proficiency in English. My second language is French, and I interpret predominantly for refugees from the African continent for whom French is their first European language. I'm thus a fly on the wall to the interactions of professionals with the users of their services. Here are two examples showing professionals who do (or don't) 'go the extra mile'.

THE CONSULTANT AND THE ADMINISTRATOR

My services had been requested by a consultant gynaecologist in an out-patients' clinic. As I sat down beside the woman for whom I had come to interpret and introduced myself, I realised that I had seen her before. It's always difficult when that happens. You talk, you try not to drop any bricks, and all the time you are trying to dig up the details in your memory.

Where was it? I'm sure she was pregnant, I thought. Yet there was no sign of pregnancy now. She had an appointment with a gynaecologist, but not in the maternity department. What had happened?

Slowly the details came back to me. The first time that I'd interpreted for Celeste (I'll call her by a fictitious name) I'd gone on a home visit with a health visitor. The interview had left me with a residue of discomfort, which is probably why I had remembered it.

Celeste was a recently arrived refugee from Africa; she and her lively four year-old son were living in temporary accommodation. The child was exuberant, but Celeste herself was quietly hesitant, impassive. She was living by herself, she said. She was possibly shy, possibly traumatised.

The health visitor ran through a list of questions about the child's medical history. Questions about the child's father (his family's medical history) met with reluctance, a shaking of shoulders, a stonewalling, yet the health visitor persisted with all the sensitivity of an elephant in an NHS uniform. I felt distaste at being obliged to relay her questions. I wanted to remind the health visitor that she was speaking to a refugee. Did she have any comprehension of the kind of experiences that might have driven Celeste to leave her country and seek refuge in the UK?

Now that I'd located Celeste, I felt happier, but I was still troubled by an elusive memory that I had helped a midwife to book her in for a confinement. As I sat there, trying to pin down what was left of these memories, Celeste turned to me. She put her hand on her womb and said something. I hardly caught the words. I could see from the expression of suffering on her face that things had gone wrong.

And then we were called in to the consultant. She was a woman in her thirties; beside her sat a younger male colleague who seemed to be learning the ropes.

The consultant gestured to us to sit down. She explained to her colleague that the patient had come in and undergone emergency surgery, and that the baby had died.

'I'm sorry about what happened,' she told Celeste.

I was still struggling to find the appropriate words to translate this when the consultant continued with her agenda. She explained the possible reasons for the problems that Celeste had had, and told Celeste that she wanted her to come in for investigation.

Celeste was monosyllabic and uncommunicative.

The consultant took out her dictaphone. Ignoring us all, she dictated a couple of letters to colleagues requesting action. Then she gave Celeste detailed instructions of what to expect and how she was to respond.

Did Celeste have any questions?

Celeste said nothing.

'Quite honestly, I think she's still in shock at what you've just said!' I protested, but this drew no response from the consultant.

We were in and out in a little more than five minutes. Celeste looked a bit dazed, and I wasn't sure that she had retained the instructions that she had been given. I was also furious at the way that she had been treated. I motioned to her to wait while I got myself signed off. Then I patiently went through the instructions again, and apologised for the consultant's behaviour.

I was about to leave, when Celeste said:

'Would you do something for me?'

'Yes of course!' I said.

Celeste then explained that they had taken a photograph of the dead baby, but at the time she didn't want to have anything to do with it. Now she had changed her mind. They had told her that the photographs would be kept at the hospital. Could I help her to find it?

It didn't take long to locate the administrative section responsible for keeping these tragic records. Twenty minutes later, we were ushered into the office of a senior manager. She handed Celeste the photo of her dead baby.

Celeste's eyes filled up. She sat gazing at the photo, taking it in. The two of us were silent. After a pause, the manager remarked how upsetting it was when something like this happened. Did Celeste have anyone to talk to? I translated for her.

Celeste shyly shook her head.

Would she like to have someone to talk to?

By the time we left, a referral for counselling had been made.

THE GENERAL PRACTITIONER

She was a refugee from a troubled African country. She had been here a couple of years or so. She went to the GP with a complaint about pain in her elbows and pain in her ankles. He made a diagnosis, suggested treatment. Told her to come back after a while.

She tried the treatment, but there was little improvement. Something different was suggested. Again she came back. Was given something, and told to come back if it didn't work. Each time, there was an interpreter because she didn't speak much English. I was the interpreter on the first occasion.

As luck happened, she was seen by one of the other doctors in the practice on her subsequent, third visit. I was once again the interpreter. The doctor pursued the outcomes of the treatment that his colleague had offered. Then he said thoughtfully:

'Are you under any stress at home?'

Yes, there was stress, she admitted. She wasn't very forthcoming about it, and the doctor could have left it at that. But he persevered with his questions.

'What kind of stress?'

Housing and financial.

'Anything else?'

She doesn't sleep very well, she said.

Again, that could have been the end of the matter, but the doctor, a gentle and sensitive practitioner, wasn't satisfied. 'Have you got things on your mind, things that worry you?' he asked.

Little by little he drew out a horrific tale of murder, rape, and eventual escape from a war-torn country. At last, he suggested that the complaint that she'd come to discuss was the least of the problems facing her, and offered to refer her to specialised services for the victims of war.

As I left the surgery, I felt privileged to have been part of such impressive professional service. Sadly, it's all too rare.

FORTY-FIVE

THE SOUND BARRIER

Michael Simmons

Long before deafness came to me – during adolescence, in fact – one of my favourite poems was Siegfried Sassoon's 'Everyone Sang'. It's opening lines almost startled me when I first read them: 'Everyone suddenly burst out singing; And I was fill'd with such delight'. They seemed to say all there was to be said about the unique and unexpected joy that the sounds of music can bring; specifically about the joy of unaccompanied voices singing spontaneously together. It was only much later that I became aware of Sassoon's deep and festering anger and bitterness about the war in which he fought and which possessed him until the day he died, nearly 50 years after it had ostensibly finished.

When I was about the same age as that young poet had been, I was seized by the scruff of the neck, as it were, on first hearing the amazing, hair-raising sounds of Beethoven's Choral Symphony, and astonished, some years later, to learn that they had, in fact, been produced by this cantankerous old man (a little over 50 at the time!), who was actually *deaf*. Poor, poor man, I thought, that he never heard his own work, and this work in particular.

The music of words and of music itself had always had charms – ever since I first heard Vaughan Williams' 'Overture to The Wasps', on a lunchtime concert of the old BBC Home Service, and, soon afterwards, Rimsky-Korsakov's suite 'Scheherezade', at a concert given by a visiting orchestra in the odd setting of the Spa Hall, Scarborough, which I, then a schoolboy, had slipped into on the off-chance. The singing of birds, too, had always had a perennial fascination. It was to be a source of rich amusement to my two sons, when they were teenagers with very different

Source: *Guardian* 14 September 2002. Reproduced by permission.

musical and other preferences, that I bought a gramophone record – the latest in technology then, you understand – of English birds.

This quite unexceptional wistfulness has been occasioned by the fact that in the past few years I have found myself joining the steadily growing ranks of the nearly nine million people in Britain who are either deaf or hard of hearing. Half a dozen or so years ago, in the final phase of a career as a journalist, I found that I was increasingly having to lean forward to hear the words of the person sitting at the next desk, that I was not always catching first time something vital that my wife, or the shopkeeper, or the bus conductor, or anyone else, had to say to me.

There was a spasm of panic at the time, but it was somehow pushed away. But then, as with so many people in a similar situation, coping with incidental one-to-one conversations in a crowded room suddenly rather than gradually became difficult. Despite their innate pleasurable qualities, these conversations started to become something I began discreetly avoiding, if at all possible. I was aware of an unfamiliar sense of creeping isolation: little bits of the fabric of life were quietly falling away.

Excursions into tinnitus – the buzzing, ringing or hissing, or other sounds that do not come from an identifiable external source – can be plain irritating, though there is the consolation, if that is the right word, that plenty of people make these excursions, just as plenty of people catch colds or get insect bites. Tinnitus can often be treated. But the journey into deafness, or into hard-of-hearingness, can be one of the most painful and sad that one can make. The euphemism seems to be that one has hearing 'impairment', a word which has its own soothing political correctness – but which does nothing whatsoever to relieve the pain. The bear with a sore head still has a sore head.

It is the obligatory, the all-consuming and the inevitably repetitious nature of the journey that is so unexpected. Deafness, especially when it comes to older people, can of course be 'eased' by some of the marvels of modern electronic technology, but the stark truth is that it is also irreversible. Every day it is there; every day the grappling with everyday sounds, however minimal, is resumed; every day, if one is used, the hearing aid, usually a flesh-coloured lump of plastic, is to be shoved into the ear and adjusted; every day the silly little battery has to be checked to ensure it has enough life to sustain the connection with the outside world. At least a pair of specs, if they sit comfortably on the nose and have been accurately prescribed, can give 'normal' sight. It is a mark of the 'naturalness' of specs that you can storm round the house looking for them, when all the time they are, literally, right before your eyes, where they were made to be.

Hearing aids can be, of course, wonders in their own right, but, in my experience, they have none of the outward normalcy or 'naturalness' of glasses. For a start, once you start wearing one, you are constantly aware that you have what might as well, for all its good intentions, be a blob of cotton wool in your ears, or you feel rather as you might when sitting in an aircraft towards the end of a flight at that moment when the change of air pressure unblocks the ears. The feeling of release when the aid is removed, however, although paradoxically all sound is once again muffled, can be as refreshing as a summer breeze. The joy of going for a swim, when the aid must be removed, is intensified.

When you turn on the aid, there is always sound. If I use the device that I was given after tests with the NHS, I am constantly accompanied, as I walk along the street, by the sound of a non-stop express train rushing by in the middle distance. Every sound – and I mean every single sound – is amplified and you can not, as you can without such a device, listen selectively. The everyday sound of, say, the rustling of newspaper pages being turned can be deafening; the clatter of saucepans or of a chair being moved across a vinyl floor can be, well, deafening. On the other hand, the car bearing down on you as you seek to cross a busy road may not be heard at all. At best, the new sounds are merely different; at worst, hopelessly distorted.

Adjusting the aid is not like turning up the volume of the TV or CD player, where the actual quality of the sound remains roughly the same. With a hearing aid, it seems rather like the opposite of fine-tuning. The nice newscaster is no longer speaking his or her words, but shouting them. Reaching a compromise with a normal-hearing companion who is in the room at the same time can be tricky. Perhaps, with practice, things will get better. Perhaps.

But not in all areas. Entering a crowded auditorium or restaurant must be the nearest one gets to incipient pandemonium, and then even carrying out the requisite double clicking on the aid to obliterate background noise is inconsistent in its effectiveness. The ambience, after all, of every auditorium and every restaurant, like the indefinable sense of expectation, is different. Then there is the erstwhile joy of walking along, say, breezy clifftops. If you have the aid on, you are assailed for the duration by a harsh sound that resembles someone next to your head constantly tearing canvas; if you turn it off for relief, then you can have no serious conversation with your companion.

Some will point to what is mysteriously known as the 'redundancy factor'. This is what comes into play when it is alleged that people who are 'hard of hearing' don't listen enough, that they make do and somehow get by on roughly 40% of the conversation going on around them. It is suggested that they learn their own 'tricks', such as putting in an odd interjection here or there, or offer a token reactive facial expression, all giving the impression that they are participating, when in fact they're clutching desperately at straws. Maybe. But the other side of the same coin is that 60% of the same thrilling – or boring – conversation may be lost. And 60% if you are in sought-after and/or congenial company, or if you enjoy, or have in your time enjoyed, good conversation, is a lot to lose.

Even travel, whether at home or abroad, brings unexpected complications. An unfamiliar dialect or a strong accent of the character you meet in the market place or drinking house, which can be one of the joys of going away, can become something to worry about. It is a new slant on investing in this or that exotic holiday destination.

In the wider context, the redundancy factor has many other implications. It means, for instance, that even interesting theatres without decent acoustics, especially ones with no useful facilities (such as those head-sets that make one feel like a Wellington bomber pilot at work), become no-go areas. Concerts, open-air meetings, lectures, poetry readings, or any function in an area bigger than the average classroom, where there is no provision for faulty hearing people, can all too frequently become pointless destinations. And one added complication: in many cases, you don't know, or you momentarily forget, that you are entering a no-go area until you get there and have tried it. By then, often, it is too late and the investment, not just of time and money, but also of anticipatory wishful thinking, has been wasted.

One of the hardest things to bear is the loss of intimacy in all sorts of relationships. Understandably, one's spouse can be driven up the wall when he or she has to say again – and possibly yet again! – a sentence of little consequence. For these sentences have their own life-enhancing importance. The ones that really matter are willingly repeated for the very reason that they do matter. But it is the ones of little consequence, day-to-day asides, that have their own spontaneity and are often the bread and butter of intimate, not to say affectionate, conversation that can be difficult to say more than once. If you are hard of hearing, you learn very quickly that thoughtless chat is not at all what you might have thought it was: it is, in fact, the nitty-gritty of social relationships of all sorts. It's also the very stuff of casual exchanges at the workplace, in the pub, street and shops – all of which become casualties.

In this context, the whisper is also virtually lost – you resign yourself to the fact that you may never hear a whisper, good, bad or mischievous, ever again.

Calamities, big and small, may arise. The front doorbell or the ring of the telephone may be missed; irritating to all concerned, and also intensely isolating and demoralising for the one who misses. (Fortunately, there are amplifiers for telephones, which make them sound like a louder doorbell.) Telephone conversations, it should be added, remain pleasurable, and, as with many hard-of-hearing people, are strangely easy to manage. A little extra gentle pressure with the earpiece on the ear can work wonders.

Hearing aids come in all shapes and sizes, and at all sorts of prices. There is a rudimentary one that comes readily from the NHS and that is slung, conspicuously visible, over the 'bad' ear. But it is quite possible to spend £3,000 for a bit of plastic that goes three-quarters the way into the ear, and is much less visible – and, therefore, arguably less helpful – to the people you are with. It is always possible that when they see you are wearing an aid, they will make that extra effort. Disaster strikes if you drop the thing, get it wet (when washing, showering or shaving, or simply walking through heavy rain) or, worse, if you mislay or lose it. But, of course, the insurance company leaps in with an offer to up the annual premium to take care of these things.

Worst of all, it can go wrong. My present aid, made by an Austrian company, cost me £1,400, after a 10% reduction because I was an oldie. As soon as I started using it, there was the excitement of hearing some birdsong again, of hearing 'normal' conversation in the sitting room, or even a quiet restaurant or similar. But within a fortnight I was back with my supplier because it had ceased to work, because – he told me – the little hole that mattered was bunged up with wax. Then, after a few months, I was back again because it had packed up altogether and made strange rattling sounds when it was gently shaken. It had to be returned to the manufacturer, and I was without it for seven days, with no compensatory replacement while it was being repaired, except my own antediluvian NHS thing, which, fortuitously, I had not thrown away. Courtesy cars at the garage there may be during a guarantee period; courtesy ears there are not.

But even in a life with new dimensions of loneliness, there are compensations. You know all the time that you are not getting the complete aural picture, and that is saddening; but you have some new joys as well. Dreams, for instance, are richly enhanced, because you are not deaf in your dreams and conversational and other exchanges are, as they were once in waking, totally uncomplicated and so enjoyable to the point of being exhilarating. Reading, a solitary occupation, anyway, becomes even more pleasurable than before, and writing, which I did for a living, ever more therapeutic, as well as creatively rewarding. Even DIY and cooking bring glimpses of the possible. And while you are busy with new pursuits, there is the satisfying thought that the number of deaf and hard-of-hearing people is steadily increasing as more people live longer.

But the losses, when you stop to think about them, can hurt very much. The London suburb where I live has its own resource centre for the hard of hearing. It offers help, information and support. It is a place I am too proud to visit, but I have its telephone number at my elbow and, if real desperation strikes, I know its address. And I note particularly that it offers support. In its latest newsletter, which I picked up, I think, at the doctor's surgery, I read the following words, which, the editor said, had been sent in by a centre volunteer called Frank. They brought tears of understanding to my eyes.

> *When you impatiently say 'Never mind'*
> *I shrivel up inside.*
> *For I frantically fought to hear what you said*
> *And you don't even know I tried.*

Not Sassoon, perhaps, but very much on the ball in the sensitivity ratings.

Some things of incalculable value are lost irretrievably. Despite a frequently revived feeling of admiration for Beethoven, for Goya, for Lord Ashley (the deaf Labour peer), even, it seems, for Bill Clinton, and a host of others who have been similarly afflicted, the regrets remain. A brief anecdote may explain: 10 years ago, before my ears and the ageing process betrayed me, my wife and I were on a group holiday in Egypt. We had stopped the coach, as one does, for a few minutes on a road in the middle of the desert. It was sunset and a very beautiful moment.

Suddenly, I heard singing (and, yes, Sassoon did come to mind). The sound was of men's unaccompanied voices, rich in harmony, vigorous in tone and relishing the rhythm of the words they sang – faint at first, but drawing steadily nearer. They came abreast of us, waving and smiling, and then passed us, gradually receding towards and then beyond the opposite horizon, singing all the way. Their sounds hung in the air long after they had passed. They were building workers, or similar, in a pick-up truck, going home after a day at a big construction site down the road. Like the first time I heard the Choral Symphony, it was a moving, magical experience. But it was almost certainly unrepeatable.

FORTY-SIX

EXTRACTS FROM 'A LEG TO STAND ON'

Oliver Sacks

BECOMING A PATIENT

[...]

He arranged an ambulance, and alerted the nearest hospital, about sixty miles away, at Odda.

Shortly after I had been settled in the little ward at Odda – it was a cottage hospital, with only a dozen beds or so, and simple facilities to cover the common needs of the community – the nurse came in, a lovely creature, though indefinably rigid and graceless in her movements.

I asked her name.

'Nurse Solveig,' she replied, stiffly.

'Solveig?' I exclaimed. 'That makes me think of *Peer Gynt*!'

'*Nurse* Solveig, please – my name doesn't matter. And now, be so kind, please, and turn over. I have to insert the rectal thermometer.'

'Nurse Solveig,' I replied, 'can't you take my temperature by mouth? I am in a good deal of pain, and my damn knee will go out on me if I try to turn over.'

'I cannot help that,' she answered coldly. 'I have my orders, and I have to follow them. It is a hospital rule – rectal temperatures on admission.'

I thought to argue, or plead, or protest, but the expression on her face showed that this would be useless. Abjectly, I turned on my face, and the left leg, unsupported, fell and prolapsed excruciatingly at the knee.

Nurse Solveig inserted the thermometer and disappeared – disappeared (I timed it) for more than twenty minutes. Nor did she answer my bell, or come back, until I set up a shindy.

Source: Sacks, O. A Leg to Stand on. London: Picador, 1984. Reproduced by permission.

'You should be ashamed of yourself!' she said, as she returned, her face pink with rage.

The patient next to me, a young man quite breathless from severe asbestosis, with a good colloquial knowledge of English, whispered, 'She's a horror, that one. But the others are nice.'

After my temperature had been taken, I was carted off to have the leg X-rayed.

All went smoothly until the technician, unthinkingly, lifted up the leg by the ankle. The knee buckled backwards and instantly dislocated, and I am afraid I let out an involuntary howl. Seeing what had happened, she immediately put a hand under the knee to support it, and very gently, tenderly, lowered it to the table.

'I am so sorry,' she said. 'I didn't realise at all.'

'That's fine,' I said. 'No harm has been done. It was a complete accident. With Nurse Solveig it's deliberate.'

[. . .]

'Execution tomorrow,' said the clerk in Admissions.

I knew it must have been '*Operation* tomorrow', but the feeling of execution overwhelmed what he said. And if my room was 'Little Ease', it was also the Condemned Cell. I could see in my mind, with hallucinatory vividness, the famous engraving of Fagin in his cell. My gallows-humour consoled me and undid me and got me through the other grotesqueries of admission. (It was only up on the ward that humanity broke in.) And to these grotesque fantasies were added the realities of admission, the systematic depersonalisation which goes with becoming-a-patient. One's own clothes are replaced by an anonymous white nightgown, one's wrist is clasped by an identification bracelet with a number. One becomes subject to institutional rules and regulations. One is no longer a free agent; one no longer has rights; one is no longer in the world-at-large. It is strictly analogous to becoming a prisoner, and humiliatingly reminiscent of one's first day at school. One is no longer a person – one is now an inmate. One understands that this is protective, but it is quite dreadful too. And I was seized, overwhelmed, by this dread, this elemental sense and dread of degradation, throughout the dragged-out formalities of admission, until – suddenly, wonderfully – humanity broke in, in the first lovely moment I was addressed as myself, and not merely as an 'admission' or *thing*.

Suddenly into my condemned cell a nice jolly Staff-Nurse, with a Lancashire accent, burst in, a person, a woman, sympathetic – and comic. She was 'tickled pink', as she put it, when she unpacked my rucksack and found fifty books and a virtual absence of clothes.

'Oh, Dr Sacks, you're potty!' she said, and burst into jolly laughter.

And then I laughed too. And in that healthy laughter the tension broke and the devils disappeared.

As soon as I was settled in, I was visited by the Surgical Houseman and Registrar. There were some difficulties about 'the history', because they wanted to know the 'salient facts', and I wanted to tell them everything – the entire story. Besides, I wasn't quite certain what might or might not be 'salient' in the circumstances.

They examined me as best they could with a cast. It seemed to be no more than an avulsed quadriceps tendon, they said, but complete examination would only be possible under general anaesthesia.

'Why general?' I asked. 'Couldn't it be done under spinal?'

For then I could *see* what was happening. They said, no, general anaesthesia was the rule in such cases, and besides (they smiled) the surgeons wouldn't want me talking or asking questions all through the operation!

I wanted to pursue the point, but there was something in their tone and manner that made me desist. I felt curiously helpless, as with Nurse Solveig in Odda, and I thought: 'Is *this* what "being a patient" means? Well, I have been a doctor for fifteen years. Now I will see what it means to be a patient.'

I was exaggeratedly upset. As soon as I thought about it, I recognised it readily. They hadn't meant to sound inflexible or peremptory. They seemed pleasant enough, in an impersonal way: doubtless they lacked authority in the matter; I would do my best to ask my surgeon in the morning. They had said that my operation was scheduled for 9.30, and that the surgeon – a Mr Swan – would look in to see me first for a chat.

I thought, 'Damn it, I hate the idea of being put under, and relinquishing consciousness and control.' Besides, more important, my entire life had been directed towards awareness and observation – was I to be denied the opportunity of observation *now*?

[. . .]

A little after nine, the physiotherapist came in, a powerful hockeyish woman with a Lancashire accent, accompanied by an assistant or student, a Korean girl with demure, downcast eyes.

'Dr Sacks?' she roared, in a voice as might carry across an entire field.

'Madam!' I said quietly, inclining my head.

'Happy to meet you,' she said, somewhat less loudly, giving me her hand.

'Happy to meet *you*,' I replied, somewhat less softly, giving her mine.

'How's the old leg? How's it feeling? Probably hurts like Billy-O, what?'

'No, doesn't hurt much now – just an occasional flash. But it seems sort of funny – not working right.'

'Mmm!' she harrumphed, considering for a moment. 'Well, let's have a look, and get down to work.'

She pulled back the sheet, revealing the leg, and as she did so I saw a sudden startled look on her face. It was instantly replaced by a serious, sober expression of professional concern. She seemed, all of a sudden, less bouncy, more subdued and methodical. Taking out a tape measure, she measured the thigh and then, for comparison, the good side. She seemed disbelieving of the measurements, and repeated them again, throwing a brief glance at the silent Korean.

'Yes, Dr Sacks,' she said at last. 'You've got quite a bit of wasting – the quadriceps down seven inches, you know.'

'That sounds a lot,' I said. 'But I suppose it atrophies pretty quickly from disuse.'

She seemed relieved at the sound of the word 'disuse'. 'Yes, disuse,' she muttered, less to me than herself. 'I'm sure it can all be explained by disuse.'

She put down her hand again, and palpated the muscle, and again I thought I saw a startled and disturbed look, and even a trace of unguarded disgust, as when one touches something which is unexpectedly soft and squirmy. Seeing this expression – which was, again, effaced in an instant, and replaced by a bland professional look – all my own fears, suppressed, came back redoubled.

'Well,' she said – and again that over-loud hockey-field voice. 'Well,' she bellowed, 'enough of all this – feeling, measuring, talking, and what-not. Let's *do* something.'

'What?' I asked, mildly.

'Contract the muscle – what do you think? I want you to tense the quad, on this side – don't need to tell you how. Just tense the muscle. Firm it up now – firm it up right under my hand. Come on, you're not trying. Do it with this one.'

Instantly and powerfully I tensed the quad, on my right. But there was no trace of tensing, no firming up, when I tried on the left. I tried again – and again, and again – without result.

'I don't seem to be very good at this,' I said in a small voice.

'Don't be discouraged,' she roared. 'There's lots of different ways. A lot of people find tensing – isometric contraction – tricky. One needs to think of a movement, not a muscle. After all, people move, they *do* things, they don't tense their muscles. Here's your patella – right under the cast.' She rapped the cast with her strong fingers and it emitted an odd chalky, inorganic sound. 'Well, just pull it towards you. Pull your knee-cap right up – you'll have no difficulty now the tendon's been fixed.'

I pulled. Nothing happened. I pulled again, and again. I pulled till I was grunting and panting with exertion. Nothing happened, nothing whatever, not the least shiver or quiver of movement. The muscle lay motionless as a deflated balloon.

The physiotherapist was beginning to look flustered and frustrated, and said to me severely, in her games-mistress voice: 'You're not trying, Sacks! You're not really trying!'

[. . .]

'Miss Preston,' I said, glancing at her name-tag (I had only thought of her as 'the physiotherapist' up to this point). 'I think you are talking very good sense indeed and I wish more doctors thought as you do. Most of them have got their heads in a cast' – and now it was my turn to rap the chalky cylinder for emphasis – 'but coming back to me, what shall I try now?'

'I'm sorry,' she said. 'I got carried away . . . Let's have another go. It's all plain sailing once the muscle gets going. One little contraction – that's all you need – it's that first little twitch, and then you go from there. I'll tell you what' – here her voice became sympathetic and friendly – 'I was just supposed to do isometrics with you today, but it's very important you have a success. I know how upsetting it is to keep trying – and fail. It's very bad to end up with a miserable sense of failure. We'll try *active* contraction – and something you can see. They don't want you lifting your leg, but I'll take all the weight. I'm going to lift your left leg nice and gently off the bed, and all you do is join in and help me . . . We have to get you sitting up a bit.' She nodded to the young Korean student, who bolstered up the pillows until I was in a sitting position. 'Yes, that should bring in the hip-flexor action nicely. Ready?'

I nodded, feeling Yes, this woman understands, she'll help me get it going if anyone can, and prepared myself for an almighty effort.

'You don't have to brace yourself like that,' laughed Miss Preston. 'You're not trying for one of your weight-lifting records. All you do, now, is to lift up with me . . . Up, up . . . Do it with me . . . Just a little bit more . . . Yes, it's coming now . . .'

But it wasn't coming. It didn't come, nothing came at all. And I could see this in Miss Preston's face, as I saw it with the leg. It was a dead-weight in her hands – without any tone or motion or life of its own – like jelly, or pudding, packed in a cast. I saw my own concern and disappointment writ large, undisguised, on Miss Preston's face, which had lost its façade of professional indifference, and become alive and open, transparent and truthful.

'I *am* sorry,' she said (and I knew she was sorry). 'Perhaps you didn't quite get it that time. Let's try again.'

We tried, and tried, and tried, and tried. And with each failure, each defeat, I felt more and more futile, and the chances of success seemed smaller and smaller, and the sense of impotence and futility grew stronger and stronger.

'I know how much you're trying,' she said. 'And yet, it's like you're not trying at all. You put out all this effort – but somehow the effort isn't managing to *do* things.'

This was very much what I felt myself. I felt the effort diffuse uselessly, unfocussed, as it were. I felt that it had no proper point of application or reference. I felt that it wasn't really 'trying', wasn't really 'willing' – because all 'willing' is willing *something*, and it was precisely that something which was missing. Miss Preston had said, at the start of our session, 'Tense the quad. I don't need to tell you how.' But it was precisely this 'how', the very idea, which was missing. I couldn't think how to contract the quadriceps any more. I couldn't 'think' how to pull the patella, and I couldn't 'think' how to flex the hip. I had the feeling that something had happened, therefore, to my power of 'thinking' – although only with regard to this one single muscle. Feeling that I had 'forgotten' something – something quite obvious, absurdly obvious, only it had somehow slipped my mind – I tried with the right leg. No difficulty at all. Indeed I didn't *have* to 'try' or 'think'. No effort of willing or thinking was needed. The leg did everything naturally and easily. I also tried – it was Miss Preston's last suggestion – 'facilitation' she called it – to raise both legs simultaneously, in the hope that there might be some 'overflow' or 'transfer' from the good side. But, alas, not a trace! No 'facilitation' whatever!

After forty minutes, then, which left both Miss Preston and me exhausted and frustrated, we desisted, and let the quad be. It was a relief to both of us when she went over the other muscles in the leg, having me move my foot and toes, and other movements at the hip – abduction, adduction, extension, etc. All of these worked spontaneously, instantly, and perfectly, in contradistinction to the quadriceps, which worked not at all.

The session with Miss Preston left me pensive, and grim. The strangeness of the whole thing, and the foreboding I felt – which I had managed to 'forget' the previous day, though it returned in my dreams – now hit me with full force, and could no longer be denied. The word 'lazy', which she had used, struck me as silly – a sort of catchword with no content, no clear meaning at all. There was something amiss, something deeply the matter, something with no precedent in my entire experience. The muscle was *paralysed* – why call it 'lazy'? The muscle was toneless – as if the flow of impulses in and out, such as normally and automatically maintain muscle tone, had been completely suspended. The neural traffic had stopped, so to speak, and the streets of the city were deserted and silent. Life – neural life – was suspended for the moment, if 'suspended' was not itself too optimistic a word. The muscles relax during sleep, especially deep sleep, and the neural traffic lessens, but never comes to a halt. The muscles keep going night and day, with a vital pulsation and circulation of minute impulses, which can be awakened, at any moment, into full activity.

[. . .]

Swan neither looked at me nor greeted me, but took the chart which hung at the foot of my bed and looked at it closely.

'Well, Sister,' he said, 'and how is the patient now?'

'No fever, now, Sir,' she answered. 'We took the catheter out on Wednesday. He is taking food by mouth. There is no swelling of the foot.'

'Sounds fine,' said Mr Swan, and then turned to me, or, rather, to the cast before me. He rapped it sharply with his knuckles.

'Well, Sacks,' he said. 'How does the leg seem today?'

'It seems fine, Sir,' I replied, 'surgically speaking.'

'What do you mean – "surgically speaking"?' he said.

'Well, umm –' I looked at Sister, but her face was stony. 'There's not much pain, and – er – there's no swelling of the foot.'

'Splendid,' he said, obviously relieved. 'No problems then, I take it?'

'Well, just one.' Swan looked severe, and I started to stammer. 'It's ... it's ... I don't seem to be able to contract the quadriceps ... and, er ... the muscle doesn't seem to have any tone. And ... and ... I have difficulty locating the position of the leg.'

I had a feeling that Swan looked frightened for a moment, but it was so momentary, so fugitive, that I could not be sure.

'Nonsense, Sacks,' he said sharply and decisively. 'There's nothing the matter. Nothing at all. Nothing to be worried about. Nothing at all!'

'But ...'

He held up his hand, like a policeman halting traffic. 'You're completely mistaken,' he said with finality. 'There's nothing wrong with the leg. You understand that, don't you?'

With a brusque and, it seemed to me, irritable movement, he made for the door, his Juniors parting deferentially before him.

I tried to catch the expression of the team as they turned, but their faces were closed and told me nothing. Swiftly the procession wheeled from the room.

[...]

LIMBO

The *scotoma*, and its resonances, I had already experienced – frightful, empty images of nothingness, which surged, and overwhelmed me, especially at night. As a bulwark against this – I had hoped, and supposed – would come the genial understanding and support of my doctor. He would reassure me, help, give me a foothold in the darkness.

But instead, he did the reverse. By saying nothing, saying 'Nothing', he took away a foothold, the human foothold, I so desperately needed. Now, doubly, I had no leg to stand on; unsupported, doubly, I entered nothingness and Limbo.

The word 'hell' supposedly is cognate with 'hole' – and the hole of a *scotoma* is indeed a sort of hell: an existential, or metaphysical, state, indeed, but one with the clearest organic basis and determinant. The organic foundation of 'reality' is removed, and to this extent one falls into a hole – or a hell-hole, if one permits oneself consciousness of this (which many patients, understandably, and defensively, do not do). A *scotoma* is a hole in reality itself, a hole in time no less than in space, and therefore *cannot* be conceived of as having a term or ending. As it carried a quality of 'memory-hole', of amnesia, so it carries a sense of timelessness, endlessness. The quality of timelessness, Limbo, is inherent in *scotoma*.

This would be tolerable, or more tolerable, if it could be communicated to others, and become a subject of understanding and sympathy – like grief. This was denied me when the surgeon said 'Nothing', so that I was thrown into the further hell – the hell of communication denied.

This is the secret delight, the security of Hell [the Devil says, in *Dr Faustus*] that it is not to be informed on, that it is protected from speech, that it cannot be made public ... Soundlessness, forgottenness, hopelessness, are poor weak symbols. *Here everything leaves off* ... No man can hear his own tune.

A sense of utter hopelessness swept over me.

I felt myself sinking. The abyss engulfed me. Although *scotoma* means 'shadow' or 'darkness' – and this is the usual symbolism of horror and death – I was sensorially and spiritually more affected by silence. I kept reading *Dr Faustus* at this time, especially its passages on Hell – and Music. 'No man can hear his own tune', on the other hand; on the other the noise, the infernal din of Hell. And this was literalised in the roomless room, the cell, where I lay, in the privation of music, and the pressure of noise. I yearned – hungrily, thirstily, desperately – for music, but my rotten little radio could pick up almost nothing, the building, the scaffolding, almost barring reception. And, on the other hand, there were pneumatic drills the whole day, as work was done on the scaffolding a few feet from my ears. Outwardly, then, there was soundlessness and noise, and inwardly, simultaneously, a deadly inner silence – the silence of timelessness, motionlessness, *scotoma*, combined with the silence of non-communication and taboo. Incommunicable, *incommunicado*, the sense of excommunication was extreme. I maintained an affable and amenable surface, while nourishing an inward and secret despair.

'If you stare into the abyss,' wrote Nietzsche, 'it will stare back at you.'

The abyss is a chasm, an infinite rift, in reality. If you but notice it, it may open beneath you. You must either turn away from it, or face it, fair and square. I am very tenacious, for better or worse. If my attention is engaged, I cannot disengage it. This may be a great strength, or weakness. It makes me an investigator. It makes me an obsessional. It made me, in this case, an *explorer* of the abyss ...

I had always liked to see myself as a naturalist or explorer. I had explored many strange, neuropsychological lands – the furthest Arctics and Tropics of neurological disorder. But now I decided – or was I forced? – to explore a chartless land beyond the reach of all charts. The land which faced me was No-land, Nowhere.

All the cognitive and intellectual and imaginative powers which had previously aided me in exploring different neuropsychological lands were wholly useless, meaningless, in the Limbo of Nowhere. I had fallen off the map, the world, of the knowable. I had fallen out of space, and out of time too. Nothing could happen, ever, any more. Intelligence, reason, sense, meant nothing. Memory, imagination, hope, meant nothing. I had lost everything which afforded a foothold before. I had entered, willy-nilly, a dark night of the soul.

This involved, first, a very great fear. For I had to relinquish all the powers I normally command. I had to relinquish, above all, the sense and affect of *activity*. I had to allow – and this seemed horrible – the sense and feeling of *passivity*. I found this humiliating, at first, a mortification of my self – the active, masculine, ordering self, which I had equated with my science, my self-respect, my mind. And then, mysteriously, I began to change – to allow, to welcome this abdication of activity. I began to perceive this change on the third day of Limbo.

To the soul, lost, confounded, in the darkness, the long night, neither charts, nor the chart-making mind were of service. Nor, indeed, was the *temper* of the charter – 'strong masculine sense ... enterprise ... vigilance and activity' (as a contemporary wrote of Captain Cook). These active qualities might be valuable later, but at this point they had nothing to work on. For my state in the dark night was one of passivity, an intense and absolute and essential passivity, in which action – any action – would be useless and distraction. The watchword at this time was 'Be patient – endure ... Wait, be still ... Do nothing, don't think!' How difficult, how paradoxical, a lesson to learn!

> Be still, and wait without hope
> For hope would be hope of the wrong thing; wait without love
> For love would be love of the wrong thing ...
> Wait without thought, for you are not ready for thought ...
>
> (Eliot)

[...]

CONVALESCENCE

'Why do you walk as if there were no knee? It is partly habit – this is how you walked with the cast – partly, I think, because you have "forgotten" your knee, and can't *imagine* what using it is like.'

'I know,' I said. 'I feel that myself. But I can't seem to use it in a deliberate way. Whenever I try, it feels awkward, I stumble.'

He thought for a moment. 'What do you like doing?' he continued. 'What comes to you naturally? What is your favourite physical activity?'

'Swimming,' I answered, with no hesitation.

'Good,' he said. 'I have an idea.' There was a half-smile, somewhat impish, on his face. 'I think your best plan is to go for a swim. Will you excuse me for a minute? I have a phone call to make.'

He came back in a minute, the smile more pronounced.

'A taxi will be here in five minutes,' he said. 'It will take you to a pool. I'll see you at the same time tomorrow.'

The taxi arrived, and took me to the Seymour Hall Baths. I rented a towel and trunks, and advanced tremblingly to the side. There was a young lifeguard there, lounging by the diving board, who looked at me quizzically and said, 'Why, what's the matter?'

'I've been told I ought to take a swim,' I said. 'The doctor told me, but I'm disabled. I've had surgery, I'm sort of scared.'

The lifeguard unwound himself, slowly, languidly, leaned towards me, looked mischievous and suddenly said 'Race you!', at the same time taking my stick with his right hand and pushing me in with his left.

I was in the water, outraged, before I knew what had happened – and then the impertinence, the provocation, had their effect. I am a good swimmer – a 'natural' – and have been since childhood – from infancy, indeed, for my father, a swimming-champ, had thrown us in at six months, when swimming is instinctual and doesn't have to be learnt. I felt challenged by the lifeguard. By God, I'd show him! Provocatively he stayed just a little in front of me, but I kept up a fast crawl for four Olympic lengths, and only stopped then because he yelled 'Enough!'

I got out of the pool – and found I walked normally. The knee was now working, it had 'come back' completely.

When I saw Mr W.R. the next day, he gave a big laugh and said 'Splendid!'

He asked me the details, I told him and he laughed even more.

'Good Lad!' he said. 'He does it just the right way.'

I realised then that the whole scene, the scenario, was *his* doing, *his* suggestion – that he had *told* the lifeguard precisely what to do. I burst out laughing too.

'Damnedest thing,' he said. 'It always seems to work. What one needs is spontaneity, to be *tricked* into action. And you know,' he leaned forward, 'it's the same with a dog!'

'A dog?' I repeated, stupidly blinking.

'Yes, a dog,' he replied. 'It happened with mine – Yorkshire terrier, sweet bitch, broke her silly leg. I set it, it healed perfectly, but she'd only walk on three legs – kept sparing the broken one, had forgotten how to use it. It went on for two months. She *wouldn't* walk properly. So I took her down to Bognor, and waded out to sea, carrying this stupid sweet animal with me. I took her out as far as I could, and then dumped her in and let her swim back. She swam back with a strong symmetrical paddle, and then scampered off along the beach on *all four legs*. Same therapy in both cases – unexpectedness, spontaneity, somehow evoking a natural action.'

I was delighted with this story, and with Mr W.R. generally. I was rather pleased to be compared with a dog – I much preferred it to being called 'unique'. And it brought home something about the elemental nature of the animal soul and animal motion, and about spontaneity, musicality, animation.

FORTY-SEVEN

'I MUSTN'T TELL ANYONE. BUT HE DID HURT ME, MUM'

Anne McDowall

Disabled children are three times more likely to be abused or neglected than able-bodied children, according to the most recent major study of this subject, which was done in the United States. Three times more. This should ring alarm bells right through our Departments of Health and Education and all the policy-making quangos, but it isn't.

Rarely are disabled children more than a footnote in important guidance papers. The Department of Health does not require child protection registers to identify whether children they list have disabilities. If this was done, at least we'd know how many are on the register, in what way they were abused and what action was taken. There also needs to be a major piece of research, equivalent to that in the US.

Another problem is that if children can't speak for themselves – using oral speech – they're not seen as credible witnesses.

The Council for Disabled Children and the NSPCC have convened a new body, the National Working Group on Child Abuse and Disability, bringing together a range of people with experience of the issues and a will to do something about them. My hope is that this group will achieve recognition at the highest levels and will stimulate change in the legal and care systems, as well as properly funded research.

Doreen Williams on the abuse of her stepdaughter, an adult with the mental age of a child. All names are fictitious save those of Mrs Williams and the care volunteer now in jail for her daughter's rape, William 'Keith' Isaac.

Source: *Guardian* 14 January 2003. Reproduced by permission.

Our daughter Alice was living in a small residential home for people with learning disabilities, run by Stockport social services. The workers in the home were lovely. Every week or two a volunteer, Keith Isaac, collected Alice and another resident, Brian, to take them swimming. In the minibus, Isaac also brought his son, Matthew, who had Down's syndrome and lived with his parents; Alice called Matthew her boyfriend.

Keith Isaac was in his 60s. Before retiring, he'd been a care worker with mentally disabled people for years for Stockport social services. He kept in this line of activity as a Mencap charity volunteer – he was actually vice-president of the Stockport branch.

Taking the group swimming was part of his volunteer work. I said I didn't like the idea of a man taking handicapped ladies swimming; like a six-year-old, Alice would think nothing of walking out wearing nothing. Her IQ is under 50. But the social services say these volunteers are few and far between and you have to be very grateful.

After swimming, Isaac used to drop his son at home. Then he would drive with the others to the Gateway Club, which is a social club where they all had discos and things. He'd lock Brian in the minibus and tell him to clean it, while he'd take Alice and Grace – another woman they took swimming – into the club, and that's when the rapes would take place.

We think it went on for at least a year. Isaac admitted to five [instances of intercourse with Alice]. We're sure it was more. She said if she had her period on, he'd make her do other things and give her a sweet to get rid of the nasty taste. By that, you knew it was more than five times.

I've asked Alice why she didn't tell us. She said: 'He told me that if I told a soul, then he would not let me see Matthew again. I love Matthew, and I want to see Matthew. That is why I mustn't tell anyone.' But, she said, 'he did hurt me, mum.'

The only reason it ever came out is because Alice fell and hit her head. When she reported that, there were questions. Then it emerged what he'd been doing. It was horrendous.

All of a sudden Alice had a social worker, from out of the sky! And of course it snow-balled from there.

Everybody knew, except us. It wasn't till nine days later that we got a phone call, but with very little information. Social services said Alice had said: 'Don't tell mum and dad.' The main people in charge at social services wouldn't return our calls.

But once the police were in touch they were brilliant. Neil Hewitt, the detective constable doing the investigation, he would ring and keep us informed. But social services? Nothing. I haven't had one letter or one phone call from any of the management before or since the court case [in March 2002 where Isaac was sentenced to four-and-a-half years by Manchester crown court].

I want Alice to be her age, I don't want her to be a little girl. But mentally she is a little girl. How should she be treated: as an adult or a child?

One thing I would say is that in the residential homes or going out on trips, carers or escorts should always be in pairs, because even with thorough checks, people are bound to slip through the net.

This Keith Isaac, he had no record. Talking about him, someone who used to work for Stockport social services said: 'He was so respected, he did so much good work.' What do you say? Yes, great work in the Gateway Club, didn't he, with my daughter.

FORTY-EIGHT

EXTRACT FROM 'THE BROTHERS KARAMAZOV'

Fyodor Dostoyevsky

'Active love? That's another problem and what a problem – what a problem! You see: I love humanity so much that – would you believe it? – I sometimes dream of giving up all, all I have, leaving Lise and becoming a hospital nurse. I close my eyes, I think and dream, and at those moments I feel full of indomitable strength. No wounds, no festering sores could frighten me then. I could clean and bandage them with my own hands. I could nurse the sufferers and be ready to kiss their sores . . .'

'That, too, is a great deal and it is well that you should be dreaming about that and not about something else. I shouldn't be surprised if by chance you really did do some good deed.'

'Yes, but how long do you think I could endure such a life?' the lady continued heatedly and almost frenziedly. 'That's the most important question! That's my most agonizing question. I close my eyes and ask myself: how long would you be able to bear such a life? And what if the patient, whose sores you're washing, does not at once show how grateful he is to you, but, on the contrary, begins to torment you with his whims, without noticing or valuing your charitable services? What if he should start shouting at you, demanding something from you rudely or even complaining to your superiors (as often happens when people are in great pain) – what then? Will you still go on loving him? And, you know, I came with horror to the conclusion that if there were anything that could instantly damp the ardour of my "active" love of humanity, it would be ingratitude. In short, I can work only if I'm paid. I demand payment at once. I mean I

Source: Dostoyevsky, F. *The Brothers Karamazov* (transl. David Magarshack). London: Penguin Books, 1958. Reproduced by permission.

want to be praised and paid for love with love. Otherwise, I'm incapable of loving anyone.'

She was in a paroxysm of the most genuine self-castigation and, having finished, she looked with defiant determination at the elder. 'That's exactly the same sort of thing a doctor told me a long time ago,' observed the elder. 'He was an elderly and undoubtedly clever man. He spoke to me as frankly as you, though in jest, but in mournful jest. "I love humanity," he said, "but I can't help being surprised at myself: the more I love humanity in general, the less I love men in particular, I mean, separately, as separate individuals. In my dreams," he said, "I am very often passionately determined to serve humanity, and I might quite likely have sacrificed my life for my fellow-creatures, if for some reason it had been suddenly demanded of me, and yet I'm quite incapable of living with anyone in one room for two days together, and I know that from experience. As soon as anyone comes close to me, his personality begins to oppress my vanity and restrict my freedom. I'm capable of hating the best men in twenty-four hours: one because he sits too long over his dinner, another because he has a cold in the head and keeps on blowing his nose. I become an enemy of people the moment they come close to me. But, on the other hand, it invariably happened that the more I hated men individually, the more ardent became my love for humanity at large." '

PART V

WORKING TOGETHER

INTRODUCTION

Janet Seden

Working with others is not easy. Often it feels simpler and quicker to act alone. However the evidence is that service users often get a better service when individuals and agencies collaborate to meet their circumstances, considering each person's health, social and other needs together. Agencies also protect service users from abuse. But service users say they want to be seen as people first and not fitted into artificial service-led categories in order to get help. Working together has become the 'buzz' theme of health and social care services at the beginning of the twenty-first century and 'joined up thinking', 'cross-agency working', 'team work' and 'partnership' are themes that dominate social policy and government directives. If professionals collaborate they can check each others' work and evaluate their different approaches.

Working together is not just about agency partnerships. It involves communicating and relating at all kinds of levels, between individuals, groups and teams. Partnership working needs communication to be effective and clear. This part of the book includes readings that consider this theme for individuals, agencies, teams and groups. Probably no one in the health and social care sector would argue against the idea that 'relationships are at the heart of practice' or that 'working together in partnership between professionals, services, agencies with service users is a good thing', yet effective working relationships based on trust, mutual understanding and skilled communication remain elusive in practice. The readings presented here aren't another theoretical discourse on what should happen to enable people, agencies and teams to work together. Rather they are individual accounts which illuminate the many facets of the topic, each showing aspects of what to consider and examples of experiences where partnership has or has not worked.

'The reunion' by Carol Gilmore reflects the twin themes of communication between individuals and within groups. It illustrates how communications between professionals who work alongside each other can be difficult. It also shows how a group of students respond to a difficult work environment. She humorously recalls an episode from her practice experience in which 'calling out names to a crowded waiting area, dressed like a clown, seemed to be a fate worse than death'. Underneath she felt humiliated by the dominating and bullying medical pecking order of the time. She and her colleagues handled their negative feelings by bonding together in the face of adversity. At a reunion, the author meets the nurses she originally trained with after a gap of twenty years. Carol takes the opportunity to confront the past when she meets a retired senior officer and 'found the courage to tell her how destructive I had found her to be' and how she had learned from her 'how *not* to treat vulnerable people'.

Clare Hall, writing in 2002, is also struggling to build relationships and be human in the busy world of a modern hospital. Her account shows how small and detailed actions build real care into the patient's experience. 'Synapses' is an account by Russell Celyn Jones, a hospital porter, who comforts the mother of a dead child on the way to the mortuary when the medical staff are unable to do so. His narrative highlights how everyone in a care or medical setting is part of the service, something often unrecognised in team building and training opportunities. By contrast 'Michael' writes about 'a great day' when the staff and service users are able to work very constructively together. Michael has time to think and plan and to 'step ahead of the problems'. The work is active rather than reactive and engages with other people. As he says, 'interacting and being busy takes the monotony out of the chores'. In this account, there is a sense of teamwork and common purpose that enables things to run smoothly. I wonder how much team work and planning there is in the background to build up the service?

Working together in service user groups and in teams is a central part of health and care work. In 'Social possession of identity' R. D. Hinshelwood offers a theoretical perspective on the complexities of group dynamics and the interpersonal transactions that happen. He applies a psychodynamic approach to an example of the way people in groups often try to avoid difficult feelings by blaming or 'scapegoating' others. This explanation of the way people, in small and large groups in hospitals and care agencies, behave can be helpful for individuals seeking to understand and change what they observe and experience in their workplaces. Hinshelwood's ideas also shed light on the group dynamics in Carol Gilmore's account. As Hinshelwood points out, groups can assign people all kinds of social roles.

Jacqueline Spring's account of an incest survivors group describes how the women support each other to be stronger through experiencing each others' rage and pain and avoiding scapegoating each other. Other groups had failed to help precisely because their experiences were not accepted but judged or interpreted. She says that sometimes it was difficult to understand what was happening between group members but 'owning what belonged to us, with support, brought some measure of control, and this increased as we explored the extent of our anguish, and discovered at last that it was finite, and that we had survived, and could now go on to live'.

Caring work is largely undertaken in small teams led by a manager or senior practitioner. The way the team supports members or develops identity built on trust can make all the difference to the way people approach their tasks. Three readings here provide accounts of team working, each with a slightly different focus. Sue Bailey, a nurse consultant, gives an account of how to make team meetings effective.

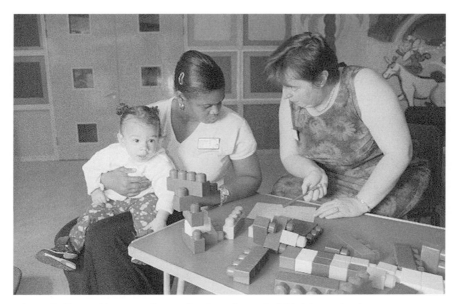

John Birdsall – Health visitor talking to family worker with child sitting on her knees.
www.JohnBirdsall.co.uk.

She argues that good communication makes room for differences to be shared openly, provided there is enough support and effective management by the team leader. This participatory style of leadership is also identified as helpful by Janet Seden in her account of 'Leadership and team culture' where she explores the team dynamics and styles of team leadership which she has experienced in social work practice environments. In 'Working with teams' Peter Miles writes as both a user of services and consultant to teams and describes himself as an 'inveterate team "watcher"'. He reflects on what he has learned about communications within and between teams. This reading also analyses those skills that can facilitate interactions between teams, agencies and services.

However hard agencies and individuals seek to work together for people who need services, it is often difficult to know where to start when you are the service user. In a second extract from her book *Remind Me Who I Am Again* (see also Part III) Linda Grant describes the minefield that exists for those relatives trying to support an elderly parent living at home. Despite the emphasis in policy guidance on 'seamless services', it is often the caring relative who becomes the co-ordinator and inter-agency broker. Often the much needed resources and services are hard to find. Fostering close working relationships between professionals and agencies means that the outcomes for service users are better and people are much more likely to get a good service. Charis Alland, in 'Ghosts in the machine', writes from experience of being a recipient of mental health services. She identifies how good communication between all the people involved is needed for someone to 'journey to recovery'.

It takes commitment, honesty, respect for others and flexibility to create channels of communication that are open and helpful. It requires a high level of ability to make relationships, build trust and communicate well to work in partnership with everyone. In the last account in this part of the book, Cicely Herbert records what it is like to be the centre of professional attention and yet to have no voice in what happens to you. It is a reminder to professionals to work together with the important person who is at the centre of their activities: the person who needs a service.

FORTY-NINE

THE REUNION

Carol Gilmore

I met a nursing colleague, Steve, again when I attended a university conference at the same site where he was the head of nursing. I rang his secretary and we arranged to meet during one of the conference breaks. It was wonderful seeing him again after over 20 years and I was as amused by him as I had always been all those years ago when we had worked together. We reflected on past times and he suggested that I attend that year's reunion at the hospital in which we had trained and I promised to think about it.

When I got home after the conference I rang Sue. She was the only person from my nursing days with whom I had stayed in close contact. I suggested that we attend the reunion – but it was a year later that we finally arranged to do so. The training had been split between two hospital sites and the reunion was due to be held in the newly upgraded one since the other hospital was now closed. We paid our £5 for afternoon tea in advance and arranged to attend for the afternoon only, missing out the formal lunch and church service. The night before, Sue stayed with me and, as we drank red wine, we reminisced about our student training days.

I recounted the story of my first day as a cadet nurse at the tender age of 16 years. It was one of the most humiliating days of my life. This was the 1960s and the era of skin-tight jumpers, the mini-skirt, stiletto-heeled pointed-toe shoes and American tan stockings. The uniform that I was given to wear on my first day was a loose, mid-calf-length daffodil yellow dress, with regulation mink-coloured stockings and black lace-up shoes that I had to provide myself. At my age and in this period this positioned me in a serious state of humiliation. I was allocated to the outpatients department, where I would work for the next 12 weeks. The senior sister in charge greeted me and showed me the waiting area and the sluice and told me to test the urine of all the new patients. I spent a terrified afternoon, dreading seeing someone I knew, during which I had to call out names, some of which I pronounced completely incorrectly. The task was made worse by the fact that I was an extremely shy person and speaking out loud was something that had been beyond my capacity at school and for which I was considered to be 'odd'. Therefore, calling out names to a crowded waiting area, dressed like a clown, seemed to be a fate worse than death.

In those days nurses outside the hospital had to wear a navy-blue mackintosh over their uniform and an outdoor hat. I had to travel home on two buses and I was convinced that everyone on each bus was making fun of me. When I got home, my mother was eager to hear every heroic detail of my first day spent 'saving lives' and 'ministering to the sick'. This was the job that she had always wanted to do and would have done so had the war not intervened. I had no time to talk to her because, not only did I feel ashamed of my first tasks, but also I was completely preoccupied with having to shorten my dresses and aprons in an attempt to regain some dignity for the following shift. My mother observed in shocked and disgusted silence as I set out to 'vandalise' hospital property. She could not understand what was wrong with this dress length, which seemed quite sensible and respectable to her.

Sue and I shared further tales of humiliation. Sue focused on the people who had made her life miserable and suggested what fate she would like them to have met. We agreed that the most common setting for humiliation was in the operating theatres. We had many tales of how the last staff member into the changing rooms had to wear the most ill-fitting clothes. For example, it was not unusual to have to wear white plimsolls or wellingtons that were two sizes too big as accessories to either a very tight and short theatre dress, or one that was voluminous and swept the floor as one walked along! This eased the task of others to be able to make fun of us temporary junior staff who had the misfortune of passing through in the guise of gaining experience. We did not feel that we had learned anything other than what fools we were considered to be. We certainly did not *see* anything – placed as we were well out of the 'action zones' in case we did any damage, the worst of which was to dirty the 'sterile field'. Making fun of any junior nurses seemed to be the main sport of the senior nursing and all medical staff. It was what might be classified as a rite of passage.

Steve had told me that the senior sister in the ENT [ear, nose and throat] theatre now worked as a volunteer in a hospice. How could she, when she had made our lives hell and intimidated staff of all categories, including consultants, for most of her working life? On my first day in ENT theatre she handed me an enormous catalogue of surgical instruments and told me to memorise the names of all the instruments displayed there – so that I could return them to their correct position in the glass instrument cupboards after the session. I could have stood there until the end of time and still not have been able to remember their names. Because of this deficit and other so-called stupid actions this seemed to seal my fate and she made my life very miserable for the rest of my 16-week allocation there. ENT theatre was worse than general theatres because only the surgeon could see what he (and they were all men) was doing, since he worked through a microscope and fiddled with grommets and such like. The report that this sister wrote of my achievement there was that I was 'kind' to all the patients. Little did she know what homicidal thoughts I harboured towards her each day as I watched the clock tick slowly through my shift.

So it was that Sue and I attended the reunion the next afternoon with mixed feelings. We were surprised to note that some of the staff on whom we had sworn revenge the night before were present. So too were those people who made life bearable and, at times, fun. At the meeting that preceded tea, one of the retired sisters read out the fate of other retired staff. This included surgeons and physicians who had worked at both hospitals. We did not entirely recognise the descriptions of their heroic devoted works. For example, could she really be describing someone whose nickname had been the 'professor of surgical complications'? One of the sisters who had died that year had actually hit a friend of mine and was being described as someone who had dedicated her life to 'caring for others'. We suppressed shock as we realised that one of Sue's wishes had come true and she was suitably contrite. It seemed to us that the death rate was unusually high. The retired sister in charge of this part of the meeting made a request for the purchase from the funds of another memorial book. Everyone agreed. It was interesting to note that record keeping was still high on the list of priorities.

At teatime, as tea was served from old metallic teapots, one of the retired nursing officers present made the mistake of asking me how I was and what my memories were of training in this hospital. I found the courage to tell her how destructive I had found her to be and how I had learned from her how *not* to treat vulnerable people. I left her in a shocked state. Sue seemed to be more preoccupied with concerns about the power of wish fulfilment and afterwards needed a lot of reassurance!

On the way home we visited the old hospital where we had done most of our training and found it to be 'for sale'. We fantasised about how we could buy it and convert it into a theme hotel. We suggested that we could wake guests up at 5.30 am, give them breakfast at 6 – unless they were 'nil by mouth' – and have all the patients sitting out of bed and their beds made by 9 am. All of the activities of the guests and any visitors could be tightly controlled by the hotel staff. These fantasies made us laugh hysterically. This is how we had always coped when we were 'in trouble'. From this shared humour we began to reduce our past fears of those powerful and unreasonable people who had controlled us and everyone else in their charge.

FIFTY

CLARE'S DAY

Clare Hall

Ward-weary auxiliary nurse Clare Hall had just one noble ambition: to comfort the sick. But in an NHS hospital, there's precious little time for caring.

I am used to the smell of death. But today it is different. The lifeless, marbled recipient of my care is a young mother. Her two young children and their father huddle distraught in the stark visitors' room nearby, trying to make some sense of what has happened. James and Kate will never see their mother again. The last memories they may have of her will be images tarnished by the barrage of equipment (tubes, wires and bleeping machines) that surrounded and engulfed her in those last few days. I have been working as an intensive-care auxiliary nurse in a large hospital for several months. My role, broadly speaking, is to provide practical and administrative support to the qualified nursing staff in their delivery of care to patients and their relatives. Nowadays, though, the work is increasingly dominated by non-clinical responsibilities; dealing with hospital waste and equipment stores, for example, along with general ward cleaning. I took the job assuming that in between the bedpans and vomit there would be the opportunity to spend personal-contact time with patients, who are often traumatised by finding themselves in an intensive-care unit. Having seen both my parents die in hospital without TLC, I believe passionately in the value of pastoral support for the recovery of the living and the dignity of the dying. So, despite being totally untrained medically, with a teaching and social work background, I threw myself in at the deep end. 'You'll receive training on the job' I was informed by the ward manager, as she thrust the crisp blue uniform into my arms and sped off to a management meeting.

Source: *Observer Magazine* 12 May 2002. Reproduced by permission.

There was to be no training 'on the job', however. Qualified staff were too busy saving lives to show a new auxiliary the ropes. Nor did I see much of the ward manager after that. I did discover the delights of bedpans and their contents, though, alone in the stifling, stomach-churning sluice – Victorian both in its archaic appearance and apparatus – where bedpans are still hand-washed with an ancient toilet brush and discarded blood bags are piled in the corner over abandoned commodes. 'Always wear gloves when touching one of those', one of the nurses warned me. Today, I am in the store-room searching for a shroud – something white as a token of respect to this young mother as she prepares for her final premature journey from this life. The porters have already wandered in to collect her, with their veiled casket. I have no time to reflect on her ultimate destination, but I do care about those she has left behind, alone and inconsolable in the visitors' room. 'We're expecting an urgent case from theatre and side room 2 needs cleaning – MRSA infection – forget anything else', Sister is suddenly barking at me and I can tell by her tone that it is pointless to argue. MRSA is the hospital superbug. Infection control takes priority over grieving relatives.

The infection-control team is due today and we must show that we are improving our performance in the battle against the bug. So I kit up, as if for bacterial warfare, before entering the infected room. The bereaved relatives are still alone in the visitors' room. No one has had time to help. A recent 'staff guidelines' pinned to the hospital noticeboard reads: 'MRSA costs the NHS £1bn a year. Nine per cent of hospital inpatients succumb to a hospital-acquired infection.' But what do these statistics, from the National Audit Office, mean to real patients? And how do you audit time taken to soothe the souls of ITU patients? Meanwhile, I need to scrub the room, bleach all visible surfaces – apparently after disinfection '16 per cent of all surfaces are still colonised' – change the curtains and await the arrival of our designated unit cleaner, who will give the floor a final 'tickle' with her special colour-coded MRSA mop. And on the ward, recently qualified nurses, their fresh young faces already etched with the stress of their job, are trying to save lives. Shadowing them constantly are the newly enlisted Filipino staff, imported to fill the gap in the labour market. There simply aren't enough nurses being trained in this country. With virtually no English, the uninitiated newcomers are still smiling naively and nodding knowingly to their tutors, but I wonder how they will communicate with frightened patients, let alone master the unintelligible medical jargon in 'Critical Care'. No one else seems to share my concern. As I slide my bleached cloth across the stained mattress, I am acutely aware that there are patients in desperate need of TLC. The tube of massage cream in my pocket hasn't been opened for days. One old lady, who has been in that bed in that corner for six long weeks now, loves having her weary shoulders and distorted feet gently rubbed; another needs her hair washed and some lipstick put on before her husband visits – 'Don't want him to remember me as decrepit,' she whispers to me one morning. An elderly man, who has no family to visit, responds with a gentle smile when you read to him. Quietly sleeping now, he hasn't been read to for days. His smile gone, the doctors are talking in guarded tones at his bedside. In contrast, Mrs Khan's extended family are always there for her. But terrified of the equipment and fearful of touching her, they need help and encouragement to hold her hand. Then there are the human resources on the unit to consider. The nurses have worked for more than six hours without a break, not even a drink. One of them keeps a forbidden can of Coke in the nurses station at the end of the bed, but it is left warm and untouched. There have been two cardiac arrests during my shift. The defibrillator, which I faithfully checked at the start of the day, has jolted at least one patient back to life: three new patients have arrived, one by helicopter. James' and Kate's mum has died, and there has been an endless stream of poker-faced consultants with their entourage of nervous doctors. An hour later and I am still cleaning: the smell of chemicals makes my eyes sore and my nose run. My hands are sweating and sticking to the Latex gloves. I stop. The room looks clean, but I am not trained as a cleaner. I came here to care. I strip off the foul, damp gloves and torn pink apron and bin them, washing my hands and smearing them with caustic alcohol gel. It should be time for a drink and I am desperate. Suffocating heat parches my throat, and there is no drinking water on the unit. 'Sorry, it's an infection risk. We can't', was the response to my request for a drinking-water machine. None of the patients has been washed yet today. Nurses are too busy checking ventilators, calculating doses of potentially lethal drugs, filling syringes, redressing leaking wounds, setting up dialysis machines, filling in forms. Always so much paperwork. 'Everything is about accountability these days', I am told more than once.

The stores have arrived and the door crashes open as large bulging wire cages are flung into the corridor. A week's supply of essential equipment is waiting to be unloaded. My back still aches from the same experience last week. Management doesn't seem to have read the recent bulletin from Occupational Health: '£2bn is lost from NHS budget annually on sick . . .' Many of these have back injuries. I am still yearning for a drink. Furtively, I head for the staff room ignoring the stores as I go. I allow my eyes to catch the pleading face of Elsie, in her late-80s, who occupies the last bed before the door. Lifting her hand to me, she mouths what was to be her final request, 'Iced water please, nurse.' In the staff room, I look longingly at the kettle and tea bags as I fill a beaker with crushed ice and collect a plastic spoon to feed her with. For a second or two I am tempted to put the neglected kettle on. Instead, I am standing with Elsie, watching the sheer joy on her face as the iced liquid soothes her moistened lips. I have forgotten the tea and I reach instead in my pocket for the cream to smooth her arthritic hands. That, after all, is what I came here to do.

FIFTY-ONE

SYNAPSES

Russell Celyn Jones

Whenever I think of a hospital I always think of it as a woman. Those sweetheart impulses governing the place are why I work here and why I never want to work anywhere else. Institutions shackle the imagination and make a stone of the heart, but this one is inspirational. It has made my luck. It's also been my longest relationship, the one anatomy I've remained faithful to, along with the women who manage my schedule: like Mavis, the control clerk who just now informs me that Patient Jackson in Cardio is awaiting a ride to Surgery One.

As I wheel a large chair out of the mess Mavis hands me a love note to deliver to the male nurse she's sweet on in Cardio. Then she starts coughing, hacking away like a plumber splitting floorboards. Sooner or later Mavis's sixty-a-day habit is going to put her on the other side of the Front Line, I keep telling her.

From the neutrality of the porters' mess I enter the stream of traumatics. Motes of dust float like spindrift in the shafts of early evening light.

In Cardio I ask the duty sister for Jackson. Without looking up from her desk she points to the far end of the ward of occupied beds, and I am as astonished by the sight of this homogenous community of the sick as on the first day I started working here, seven years ago. How it must shake you down, to be one moment pickling apricots, studying the racing form, reading an aerogramme from a prodigal child, then in the next waking up in here without use of limbs, an IV in your arm, feeding tubes up your nose, surrounded by strangers in starched white gowns. The confusion still registers on their faces.

We know them only when they are sick, but it never escapes me that these men and women, until they lost their way, have led full lives. Many

Source: Morley, D (ed.). *The Gift. New writing for the NHS*. Exeter: Stride Publications, 2002. Reproduced by permission.

of the stroke victims have lost their voices and cannot tell us these stories. So it is a matter of courtesy that they be treated with respect, as they stand naked in backless gowns, lifted on to a commode, with a raw hurt burning in their eyes. Any good medic knows to take this holistic approach – like the male nurse who helps me lift Jackson from her bed on to the chair.

I slip him Mavis's love note and can't help feeling sorry for her. Unrequited love is an illness too, with no known cure. The erotic cathexis of a hospital extends only so far. It's a doctor and nurse affair that does not engulf the auxiliary staff. On account of their quotidian contact with naked flesh, medics' desire builds throughout the day like electrons picked up by a generator. On the out, in mufti, they fall for each other. But they never fall for me, or Mavis or anyone else in the porters' mess. We are low caste, the untouchables.

The only women to fall for me have been the patients. Such as the tall Texan with psoriasis; the north London Jewish girl with diabetes; the African-American lesbian with gynaecological complications; the Irish fiddle player with cancer (God rest her soul). All these women I have had time with, but couldn't settle with any of them. They complained of me being distant, cold even. Perhaps the truth is I don't like to give out. I don't enjoy losing control, allowing someone else to push me around like the steel balls in a pinball machine. I have only ever truly belonged to one woman – my sister Geena. But that's another story.

Patient Jackson is black, in her sixties, eighteen stones on the scales and terrified. She wears a gossamer veil over her thinning hair. On her feet are slippers with little pink tassels. As I wheel her through the ward the other patients watch our progress. They can't speak and they can't raise their arms to offer her a send-off to Surgery, but I sense the goodwill in their stony silence. And gratitude in their eyes that it isn't them going under the knife.

On the way to Surgery I ask my patient what op she's having, but she doesn't reply. So I ramble on about how nice the surgeon on duty today is, which is an out-and-out lie. The surgeon's perfectly competent, but he's a racist and I know she wouldn't want to hear that. But whatever I say is lost on her. She can't speak a word of English.

In Surgery I leave the patient in a bay and go looking for a nurse. On the slab in theatre is a young woman under anaesthetic. She is having a tonsillectomy, so the surgeon really has no business peeling the sheet down to her ankles. What he is staring at with such lewd fascination is her tattoo. Her pubic bush constitutes the body of a black widow spider, its legs tattooed down her thighs. 'Can you imagine going down on *that*?' the surgeon says to me. 'One of these days some guy's going to take a two-by-four to that thing.' When I fail to reply the surgeon looks up at me, sees that I am only a porter and his eyes glaze over.

I've never wanted to be a doctor, they may perform miracles but their personalities are a disease. Men of medical science whose ambition is aimed squarely at gaining power in the institution are lost to the good world. They seek promotion, then spend their lives in politics.

I've never wanted to be a nurse either, not even a paramedic. I am happy with my place in the scheme of things. I know my Re-sus ABC, how to treat wounds, recognise dinner-fork fractures, cerebral vacuolar attacks, coronary thrombosis. These things I have picked up along the way. But I don't perform miracles. I help those who do, content with the routine that hardly changes from day to day, week to week, year to year.

Normally eight porters on each shift, we are two down today, throwing what we call a duvet-day on the busiest end of the hospital week. Which is why I am now running from Surgery into Neo-Natal, Chest, Heart, Liver and Kidney with a sack full of blood and urine samples for the Path-Lab. I am running but nurses hardly notice me. They do not care to know who I am, what I know.

The only nurses who engage with me for longer than a couple of seconds and about something other than urine samples are the West Indian mothers-of-five. They tease me in the canteen during my dinner break for having a book open on the table beside my plate. The closest they come to making a direct statement is to call me a dreamer and then throw their heads back in pearls of laughter. But in such a place as this to be a dreamer is the only way to fly.

If nurses hardly notice me the doctors don't even see me. So it comes as something of a surprise when a junior doctor sitting at my table, who has been watching me for some time with my head in my book, leans across the Formica and asks why I don't try to do something more with my life. (He is a New Zealander . . . does that explain anything?)

What is more? I ask.

He points to my book. More would be taking a degree course in the care management.

I say, When you refuse all power no one will ever be afraid of you.

The junior doctor laughs and asks why I read if not to advance myself.

I tell him, what I read and what I do for a living move in opposite directions.

The junior doctor admits that he has no time for reading, on call one hundred hours per week. I tell how my lowly, dead-end job gives me not just the time but the space to absorb what I read. The job is not who I am.

Then who are you? He wants to know.

All I know for sure is that I am a reader and that literature is as real as any hospital. He seems to think about it for a second, then replies. Work is a defence against despair.

I say, What is your defence against work?

The junior doctor gives up on me and leaves the canteen and I am able to return to my book, *All Quiet on the Western Front*, that does not flinch from describing the wounded and the dead. The characters are teenage recruits who, unlike the patients in Cardio, have not had a chance to settle into an adult life before finding themselves face-down in the earth as the darkness rocks and rages around them, as whole woods are lifted into the air and smashed to pieces. They feel a thousand years old applying emergency first aid to their school friends dying in meadows tossed like storm seas, as bayonets of even younger recruits pierce the mist of poison gas that wriggles into the trenches like jellyfish. Coffins are ripped out of a cemetery and the sky rains corpses – the dead who provide cover for the living, trying to survive someone else's bad idea.

The control clerk calls me on the shortwave and tells me to go to Thorogood Ward and take a Purple-Plus to the Mortuary. This is not as contradictory as it seems (what I read and what I do move in opposite directions, etc.). As many people come here to die as to be cured. Nonetheless, Mavis feels the need to warn me in advance that the Purple-Plus is a girl of nine, a victim of meningitis.

I can hear the wailing from outside the ward. As I enter Thorogood I see the commotion created by the mother who lays across the bed and won't allow anyone to take her child away. But there are patients waiting for this bed and two nurses are gently trying to prise the mother's hands from the body. It is very upsetting for everyone.

I suggest that I take the mother as well to the Mortuary. So she sits in my wheelchair, this poor stressed woman, and the nurses lay the corpse, wrapped in a starched white sheet, in her lap.

Outside the ward the movement of the chair seems to comfort her. There is a sense of optimism that comes from motion, as though time is somehow being reversed. She is even able to talk with me, explaining how her daughter was at a birthday party when she was taken ill. Then her grief is fully reprieved as we enter the elevator. Two other persons, laughing as we step into the lift, are immediately silenced by the tangle of bodies on my wheel chair, by the sight of five fingernails painted orange protruding from the sheet and a flash of red hair flecked with silver glitter that the mother holds in her hand.

Mavis finds me on the shortwave again while I'm still in the Mortuary. She saves me from my morbid feelings with a detail designed to give me a lift. She tells me to go and deliver a couple of oxygen cylinders to Maternity.

Maternity is the only wing of the hospital where no one is actually ill. In pain maybe, but very different to the pain in, say, Cancer or A&E. Maternity is upbeat, a gold rush town where every panhandler walks away with something precious. Five, maybe ten times a shift I go into Maternity and witness at least one child being born into the world. And sure enough, as I arrive, a girl (eight pounds, six ounces) is delivered to a bricklayer's wife, as he stands weeping with joy over her bed, raising the flag in the memory cells of the infant's brain. Synapses bring out the very best in human nature. Love is biological imperative and such intense moments of it that I see may never be achieved again. But that's the thing about Maternity, you get to see truth and beauty at its peak. So whenever my control clerk sends me to Delivery Suite, it's free air miles to me.

FIFTY-TWO

A GREAT DAY

'Michael'

Michael is a care assistant in a residential service for people with learning disabilities and autism

I drive up the steep hill to the grand old house that once was the home and the surgery of the village doctor. How sick patients ever got up there, before the days of the car, I'll never know. The house is now the home of five people with learning disabilities. Walking towards the house, I see Tom peeking out of the window, and as I go to the back door which leads to the kitchen, he is waiting there to give me a warm handshake at this the start of my shift. Tom is unable to speak so I assume this is his way of saying 'hello'. Since I started working here eighteen months ago, there has never been a day when I haven't looked forward to my day's work. Each day brings unpredictability and variety. And today, it looks as though Tom is in good form; hopefully there will be no hitting out at others today. Also in the kitchen are my two colleagues and they are busy preparing breakfast for the residents. They all greet me. One says it's great to see me; we haven't shared a shift for some time and we work very well together. I fill the kettle to make coffee for everyone there. Aisling is sat at the table after having her breakfast and I know for sure she will not refuse a cup of coffee. That is her delight and her problem. She will often drink too much and if you try to restrict her she will become aggressive. We take time to sit with our coffee and discuss what type of activities we can do in the day ahead and who will do what with whom. Because most of the people who live in this house are diagnosed with autism, we have procedures and routines that we have to stick to in order to create some predictability and consistency in their lives. Sudden change can lead to mayhem.

Sometimes things do not go according to plan; the weather, staff and resources all come into our decisions. Afterwards I go upstairs to wake Ian for his breakfast, he's a late riser. Once he is dressed, we make his bed together. Ian has rituals where he spins around as he walks. I encourage him to collect his night clothes and bring them to the Laundry Room as he spins his way to the kitchen. I then go to wake Jamie. Unfortunately Jamie wears splints on both arms almost all of the time, to prevent him from hitting his face. Changing clothes, eating, washing and some activities are the only times the splints are removed and these can be really stressful times, for him and for staff. We are working towards him spending time without splints and most evenings we try to remove them and create a relaxing atmosphere so that he can associate relaxation with removal of the splints. He seems happy today. I know this because he draws me to him to touch my face. I find it very distressing when he hits himself, it's as if it hurts me as well, and sometimes this starts first thing in the morning. So, today, finding him in a good mood makes me feel happy. I help Jamie to dress himself and to make his bed. There is a little bit of him hitting his face but we take it slowly. Afterwards he puts his night clothes into the basket and we go to the Laundry Room. On our way, we meet Pauline who is singing and clapping to music on the radio in the hallway. She's in great form today. She has a fantastic ear for music. Sometimes we use music and singing to help her calm down when she is distressed. I arrive at the kitchen along with Jamie and Pauline to join Ian, sitting at the kitchen table. Ian can at times become impatient when he requests certain items for breakfast and staff are unable to deliver as quickly as he is asking for them.

We always have to be aware of potential problems and try to prevent them happening where possible. After breakfast has finished we get down to working with residents to do the household jobs. I like this time because interacting and being busy takes the monotony out of the chores. It's a time to find out people's progress and their limits, to see if they've learned since the last time. I find that adding humour and fun makes the job twice as easy. Today Jamie and I are doing the vacuuming and I notice that he quite enjoys the movement of the vacuum cleaner and he is very thorough in carrying out the task. The weather is fine so, afterwards, we all go for a walk down that steep hill around the village, pick up a few items in the shop and back up the hill again. We return to have a quick snack and then off out shopping on the mini-bus. It's the weekend and some of the residents have gone home, so with such small numbers we go to a restaurant for a meal before our shopping. The day has been great, and gone by so quickly. We arrive back home to relax for a while. Over a cup of coffee myself and the other two members of staff allocate who is going to be responsible for what. We decide that since Jamie has been showing so little self-injury, we will minimise the amount of change for him and I will continue to work with him.

Afterwards I bring him for a bath, where I remove his splints and he immediately starts to hit his head with his arm. Once he is in his bath he starts to relax. When we arrive down to the kitchen, the staff and the others have prepared supper. After enjoying supper – we all muck in and tidy up and it's time then for residents to relax before retiring to bed for the night. Most of us congregate around the TV. It's also time for me to go off duty from my long day.

FIFTY-THREE

SOCIAL POSSESSION OF IDENTITY

R. D. Hinshelwood

The psychoanalytic concept of projective identification is a mechanism of intrapsychic defence (Klein, 1946). It is also an element in interpersonal relatedness (Ashbach and Sharmer, 1987). It is therefore one of the bridging concepts that we have between the intrapsychic and the social. There are other bridging concepts between the individual and the social, ones which come from the social sciences; in particular I will deal with 'role' (Miller and Rice, 1967; Agazarian and Peters, 1981) and 'alienation' (Geyer and Schweitzer, 1981; Meszaros, 1970).

I shall describe a process that consists of a sequence of repeated projective identification that proceeds through a network of relationships (Hinshelwood, 1982). It is as though a path can be traced from one person to another; I shall illustrate with material first from a small therapy group and then from a working institution. This process throws light on the difficult and alienating experience of being in large institutions. I shall then examine the general properties of this process and its relationship with the concepts of 'role' and 'alienation'.

A SMALL-GROUP EXAMPLE

It is a quite ordinary session of a group with five members and a therapist. At the beginning of the session it had been announced that a new member

Source: Richards, B (ed.). *Crises of the Self. Further essays on psychoanalysis and politics.* London: Free Association Books Ltd, 1989. Reproduced by permission.

would be joining the group. After an initial half an hour of discussion about one member's domineering manner of talking, she (Mrs A) became quite angry at what felt to her like criticism. She turned to Mr B, a reticent man, who had been less involved than the others and said 'Well, at least I do more than you.'

In this interaction Mrs A was justifying herself and passing on her sense of being criticized to Mr B. The insertion of her own feeling state into Mr B is a projective identification by Mrs A.

Mr B looked up rather surprised and awkwardly said that he had been thinking over, since the session last week, what had been said by Mr C who had told Mr B that his silence was a kind of dishonesty because it kept people mystified about what he was thinking and made them uncomfortable. He continued that he thought Mr C was wrong, and that there was nothing wrong with being fairly quiet. It was a question of keeping one's own privacy; one was entitled to do that. Mr C, he complained, was now pestering Mrs A in a equally unkind way. He asked, rhetorically, why could Mr C not stop getting at people.

Mr B in turn was passing on the sense of being in the wrong to Mr C.

Mr C looked around him rather startled, as he had not really been the only one tackling Mrs A on her intrusiveness. He went a little red in the face and started to justify himself on the grounds that someone in the group had to confront difficult things, but this defensiveness abruptly changed to a more hectoring quality as he began to complain that the therapist did not do these things which were so difficult for the members of the group. The therapist should control things if they went wrong. At this point the therapist suddenly felt on the spot and that he was letting the group down. He felt he had to do something to stop the nasty atmosphere that was developing in the group. Provoked in this way to do something, he came in quickly to say that Mr C was clearly seeing him (the therapist) as irresponsible. He rather clumsily related this to what the group knew about Mr C. Mr C was a rather direct man from an unsophisticated background who had come to treatment because of repeated violent episodes in pubs and finally once at work with a customer. The therapist explained that Mr C felt bad because it played on his feeling that he was a violent man.

I hope it is clear that so far there is an uncomfortable interchange going on in which Mrs A's sense of guilt or blame was transmitted first to Mr B who then tried to put Mr C in the wrong. Mr C in turn made the therapist feel guilty and irresponsible.

The therapist's hasty intervention did not alter the atmosphere significantly as it returned the focus to Mr C. Mrs A made a pun on Mr C's name (Vic) suggesting he had a violent need always to be the victor. There was laughter that relieved some tension for the members of the group, apart from Mr C who erupted with rage in a punitive outburst against the whole group. The smiles faded rapidly as an atmosphere of fear gripped the group, and Mrs D, a depressed woman, began to cry. Her crying seemed to make Mr C feel reproached even more. He seemed to be torn between hitting her and leaving the group. His control was sufficient for him to stand up and turn slowly towards the door. At this point the therapist intervened more thoughtfully and said that Mr C was needed by the rest of the group to take away from the group everybody's anger and rage at being let down. Mr C remained standing at the door for some ten minutes while the group, in fear, began slowly to pick its way consciously through what had happened. As some of the other members of the group became aware of what Mr C represented for them he was able rather sullenly to return to his place and remain a brooding presence silently reproaching the group.

The whole sequence has five steps. (1) Firstly Mrs A was put on the spot by the members of the group in order to examine an aspect of her relationship with them, her domineeringness. She began to feel to blame for what she does. (2) She then made the point that she was not as bad as someone like Mr B and thus passed on her sense of being blamed to Mr B. (3) He adeptly managed to pass it on again, this time to Mr C, blaming him for what Mr C had said the week before. (4) Mr C managed to control himself by, in turn, passing on this sense of blame to the therapist. (5) The therapist then tried to make an interpretation but was filled with the blame put into him, and succeeded only in passing the sense of blame back to Mr C. And there it rested for a while, as Mr C acted in such a way as to accrue more blame for his explosive outburst.

I am drawing attention to the way that a *feeling-state*, in this case a sense of blame, is passed on from one member of this group to the next. The process halted when one person, Mr C, came to be established as the blameworthy culprit – a scapegoat.

My thesis is that an essential ingredient of a social network is that bits of experience, affects, emotions, feeling-states, are moved around. These channels of unconscious, non-symbolic communication are separate from, but intertwined with, the verbal and cognitive communication. I will term this aspect of the network, the *affective network*.

AN INSTITUTION'S NETWORK

The other example is a set of observations from a day hospital. It shows a chain of similar emotional events (projective identifications) taking place in the affective network of an institution.

1   Dr A had advised one of his patients, Mr B, to leave the hospital and return to work, and was thus pushing him to accept that he had failed at his university career.

2   Mr B's symptoms intensified. He believed one of the occupational therapists, Miss C, was in love with him. Delusionally, a failure at university had become a success in love. When Miss C did not admit she was in love with Mr B he became abusive and threatening towards her. It was an intimidating attempt to make Miss C feel a failure – i.e., a projective identification of part of his feelings into Miss C.

3   Miss C sought support from a fellow occupational therapist, Mrs D, against the abuse from Mr B. She passed on part of her fear and intimidation to her colleague.

4   Mrs D then tackled Dr A and attacked him for not giving sufficient support to the non-medical clinical staff. Failure and blame had come around full circle to be put back to Dr A.

5   Dr A then had a further discussion with Mr B about leaving and about his abusiveness towards Miss C.

6   Following this Mr B became aggressive with other patients, throwing a piece of wood across the workshop in one of the OT sessions.

7   The effect on the patients was a paradoxical one. Mr B's violent event was a very concrete form of projecting his state of mind at the rest of the patients and occupational therapists. He frightened the others and they turned to each other for support. This took the form of another delusion intended to reassure everybody. It was asserted that the hospital was a peaceful and tranquil paradise.

The patients' view of the hospital as a soft option, a peaceful, untroubled paradise, had been a recent topic of discussion among the staff; and it seemed to them that consequently patients stayed there too long and became chronic. As a result the staff believed they should challenge the view of the hospital as paradise and introduce a stricter regime.

8   The staff then reacted by increasing their resolve to toughen up the hospital regime and new energy was put into discussing and shaping this new policy.

The affective network 'contained' the initial traumatizing of Mr B by passing on the emotional element or piece of identity (in this instance Mr B as a failed student) from one person to another. As it flowed through the network it changed – from failure, to aggression, to fear, to delusional peace, and to instituting new policies. It is of considerable interest that the initial quantum of personal experience or identity was eventually disposed of as the energy for a piece of work of the organization as a whole. It is possible to show that institutional actions are frequently driven by energy derived from the split-off parts of personal experience and personal identity.

THE PROJECTIVE LIFE OF INSTITUTIONS

There are a number of general properties of affective networks that can be seen in these two illustrations:

1 Individuals use the context of the social network as a means of passing on to others certain feeling-states, elements of identity, which they wish to disown – a form of psychological *defence by projection*.
2 Personal affects of the individuals come to be possessed by the social network to form the energy for institutional activity.

And as a result of the above two properties:

3 There is a depersonalization of the individuals' experiences and feelings.
4 The individual becomes deeply fused to the group or institution since the social network, to a degree, is the individual.

The individual becomes raw material for the developing culture, its structure and activity. His unconscious investment in it is based on primitive mechanisms involving splitting. A split piece of experience comes adrift from one member and is projected as if it were a package, a discrete quantum of experience which, in the unconscious minds of the individual members, can be taken in and given out.

The individual actually loses his own experience in the ramifications of the network and with it some of his sense of self or identity. A large institution feels inhuman because individuals literally lose themselves (or parts of themselves) in it.

Because these processes are based on the unconscious mechanisms of individuals, the institution comes to be felt unconsciously as alien, split from the individuals who make it up – 'the faceless bureaucracy', 'the monolithic organization', terms we use to convey the way institutions reduce the sense of identity of the individuals. At the same time the process binds the individual into an identification from which the individual has great difficulty in extricating himself whole.

ROLES AND THE UNCONSCIOUS

In the field of social science, roles are the collections of functions performed by the individual for the social group. Typically these roles belong to the institution but are voluntarily adopted by individuals. They can be thought about rationally and altered or adhered to for rational and conscious purposes.

However, it is not necessarily like that, since a role can be felt to be imprisoning or alienating. One reason for the imprisoning experience was shown in the example of the small therapy group arising, at the unconscious level, from projective identification. One individual came to play a specific part for the others. In that case it was a scapegoat, a well-known phenomenon that goes back to biblical times. Its relationship to widely held feelings of guilt in the group was always known too.

The precise means by which this unconscious role for the group was established is the process I have drawn attention to – a quantum of emotion, of a feeling-state or of an identity was passed around by projective identifications and finally localized in one individual who was subjected to an 'enforced introjection' (as Menzies, 1959, called it). Such a process causes the individual a distortion of his identity. Greatly enhancing certain aspects of his personality will obliterate others. At the same time, it also distorts the identity of others, depleting them of certain aspects (Hinshelwood, 1982; 1987). This unconscious function of carrying the guilt (or some other emotional aspect of identity) for the other members of a group needs to be carefully distinguished from performance of conscious, rational roles.

We need, at this point, to make some careful distinctions. A role entered into may be congenial or it may be uncongenial. Acceptance of a role may be voluntary but that does not exclude the occurrence of the processes I have discussed, in which the person in addition to his conscious role is also unconsciously elected to a position that distorts his own personal identity. A role within an identified institution may acquire specific personality characteristics through the social projective system; Menzies (1959) showed, for instance, that student nurses were regarded and treated as irresponsible without regard to their actual individual personalities, so much so, in fact, that it worked to the detriment of recruitment to the nursing service.

Also, many roles that are consciously entered into are alienating because of a specific impoverishment due to socio-economic exploitation, for example many work roles, or the role of 'mother' for some women. And many, being alienated already, may attract psychological exploitation as well: blacks may not only be correctly identified as different from whites but become stereotyped 'blacks' with anal and faecal connotations that are attributed socially but unconsciously.

The question arises of the relation between the role that is alienating because of socio-economic exploitation, and those that are so because of the psychological exploitation. In my view alienation in socially exploited roles invariably attracts exploitation for projective purposes as well, giving rise to a state of affairs in which economic exploitation and psychological exploitation go hand in hand.

Carrying a socially projected emotional identity that turns a social role into a highly restricted personality is usually felt as an alienating experience and destructive of personal development. Yet some people will take up such places that will seriously hinder their own identity development; perhaps we all do to some extent. However, it is not always consciously experienced in this way: Turquet (1975) has described advantages, as well as the threats, of a group-defined identity. Compliance with the unconscious projected identity is, at the level of the individual, akin to 'false consciousness' at the class level (Lukács, 1971). The invitation for projective exploitation is clear in the small group example, in which Mr C's emotional role, that the group needed to exploit, was close to one aspect of his personality – into which he was restricted by the group.

ALIENATION

The depersonalizing effect of projective identification at the psychoanalytic level of the individual becomes *alienation* at the level of the group network (Hinshelwood, 1983), a depersonalization of the individual actually within the institution which, to an extent, *is* him. Expropriation of a particle of his own experience comes about through transformations that occur and the individual actually loses some of his experience as it passes away through the ramifications of the network.

In our own culture the affective networks of institutions have come to be remarkably efficient at exploiting individuals' feeling-states and experiences, reifying bits of human beings and estranging them from the human world.

The affective network is an exchange system of human emotions and identity, of reified bits of human beings. In this sense affective networks parallel the exchange systems of commodities which are also reified bits of human relations. And it is possible that economic exploitation is a concrete precipitate of projective exploitation; that is to say, the projective processes are the special medium by which economic exploitation takes a hold on individuals. Capitalism has learned to accurately reflect and exploit the potential in human beings to alienate and reify qualities and identities. The way the capitalist system aligns the psychological potential for projective identification in groups and commodity fetishism in the economic system is a powerful union. To dismantle such a system requires attention to the psychology of institutions as well as the economics and politics of the capitalist system.

The losing of parts of human emotions and identity in the affective network compares with the expropriation of surplus value in the labour of economic production. Both are alienated from the individual to be exploited by the (capitalist) institution. It is likely that both 'surplus identity' and surplus value are needed in the oiling of the wheels of capital accumulation.

REFERENCES

Agazarian, Y. and Peters, R. (1981) *The Visible and Invisible Group*. Routledge.

Ashbach, C. and Sharmer, V. (1987) 'Interactive and group dimensions of Kleinian theory', *Journal of the Melanie Klein Society* 5: 43–68.

Geyer, F. and Schweitzer, D. (1981) *Alienation: Problems of Meanings, Theory and Method*. Routledge.

Hinshelwood, R. D. (1982) 'The individual in the social network', in M. Pines and J. Raphaelson, eds *The Individual and the Group*. Volume 1: *Theory*. New York: Plenum Press, pp. 469–77.

Hinshelwood, R. D. (1983) 'Projective identification and Marx's concept of man', *Int. Rev. Psycho-Anal.* 10: 221–6.

Hinshelwood, R. D. (1985) 'Projective identification, alienation and society', *Group Analysis* 18 (3): 241–54.

Hinshelwood, R. D. (1987) 'Social dynamics and individual symptoms', *International Journal of Therapeutic Communities* 8: 265–72.

Klein, M. (1946) 'Notes on some schizoid mechanisms', in *The Writings of Melanie Klein*, Volume III. Hogarth, pp. 1–24.

Lukács, G. (1971) *History and Class Consciousness*. Merlin.

Menzies, I. (1959) 'The functioning of social systems as a defence against anxiety', *Human Relations* 13: 95–121.

Meszaros, I. (1970) *Marx's Theory of Alienation*. Merlin.

Miller, E. and Rice, A. K. (1967) *Systems of Organization*. Tavistock.

Turquet, P. (1975) 'Threats to identity in the large group', in L. Kreeger, ed. *The Large Group*. Constable, pp. 87–144.

FIFTY-FOUR

SURVIVING TOGETHER

Jacqueline Spring

I drove home after my first incest survivors' group meeting, and sat for a long time in my car outside the house, trying to take in the vision I had seen for the first time that night, of the harm that incest does, the lives ruined, relationships unhappy, or broken, or impossible to undertake, survivors' children scarred, the loneliness, grief, guilt, the physical and psychological punishment meted out to victims for the rest of their lives. That I had suffered thus I knew, and had mostly come to terms with. That this same suffering had a thousand faces, a thousand variations, and yet that these variations were on the same themes, the same issues as my own, made me know that I was only beginning to see, that I had just caught my first glimpse of a boundless ocean of pain.

I was not at the group because I needed help. I was there because I felt I could give help. I didn't need help any more, I thought. I was the 'finished product'. But as we went round the group introducing ourselves, saying why we were there, it seemed that most of us were there to give help. We were all helpers, all prepared to bear each others' burdens. Perhaps bearing burdens was the only thing that we all felt qualified to do.

Hearing that many of us held the same aim as I did, made me wonder if, after all, I had come through the pain of incest. Perhaps I was fooling myself. At the time I was still mourning the loss of Eve, and that remained such a tender wound that I did not feel able to let anyone in that room touch it. Yet there was a need in me to express my loss somehow, though I didn't think that I was able to do it, that anyone in the world would be able to understand what I couldn't fully understand or accept within myself. It was this deep fear of unique pain, together with the inability to

Source: Spring J. *Cry Hard and Swim. The story of an incest survivor*. London: Virago Press, 1987. Reproduced by permission.

trust others enough to share it, that united me in spirit to the others in the group. Each of us carried many losses, sustained in many different ways. Our backgrounds, ages, educational levels, races, religious beliefs and sexual preferences varied widely, making it difficult for each of us to believe that we could all suffer in quite the same way our common tragedy. But just walking into the room that the rape crisis collective provided, into a group of incest survivors, for the first time, brought relief at the most basic level.

The simple sight of what looked a perfectly ordinary gathering of women, one that could have been picked at random from any city street, mirrored back to me, as nothing else could have, that incestuous experience had not put me at one remove from the rest of the human race. No one there was the freakish alien we had each, in our secret souls, conceived ourselves to be. This was the very first gift we gave to each other, just by sharing our physical presence.

We were there in safety, in the anonymity of first names only, to find a way to help ourselves and each other. To say where our pain was originally coming from was too difficult that first meeting, and indeed some never found the courage, or, perhaps, the need, to go into details of how they had been sexually abused. What came easier to most of us at first was to try to trace the more recent history of our search for meaning, for contact, and for healing. It was easier, but not easy.

I think of Cara, the only one of us with enough objective evidence and outside support to have been able to accuse her father in court. He had been convicted and sentenced to four years, commuted to two, for good behaviour. Two years' imprisonment for seven years of incestuous abuse, starting when Cara was ten. While he was inside, Cara had had a few meaningless cosy chats with a social worker, a full year after the court case. That was all. Cara had, with huge effort, gained qualifications to get a job within those two years, so that she could be independent, and wouldn't have to be at home when he came out, untreated and unchanged.

I think of Pat, so young, and recently escaped from her violent stepfather, rehoused in a tiny flat perched in the top corner of a vast, bleak, multi-storey building, with dizzying balconies overlooking the sprawling acres of the city, though she was known to be suicidal.

I think of gentle Susan, whose voice was almost breaking as she told of the hospital where she had spent hours every day in a huge mixed patients therapy group of men and women, impassively expected to bare her soul in front of men who were quite unrestrained in their coarse comments about women, whose use of art therapy was brazenly pornographic.

I think of Joanne, standing in front of the Children's Panel at the age of fourteen, caught for persistent truanting and running away from home. Of her fine scorn for the gentleman behind the desk, who kept reproaching her for running away – 'when you come from such a good home'.

I think of Julie, who believed in being honest, and who tried with all her might to trust her psychiatrist, telling him that she had found some comfort in her father's caresses, that he had been the only one in her environment who had cared for her. I think of how this precious, most timid admission was used to hound her for months, to pressure her into confessing that she had deliberately set out to seduce her own father.

I think of Maria, whose sympathetic psychologist sits on the other side of a desk taking notes while Maria talks, how this has gone on for years without either of them realising the stalemate that the notebook, and the necessity for it, represents.

I think of Jean saying that she couldn't come back to the group, that she couldn't bear to fathom at last the full extent of everything that has happened to her, that she couldn't stand to hear the pain of her own life story echoed back to her in the words of the other survivors talking about theirs. Tragedy heaped upon tragedy over the years, leaving her alone and finally understanding the huge weight of retribution that has fallen upon her for having been a little girl who didn't know how to refuse her father. Jean, who has never had anyone to help her through, and who did come back nonetheless, sensing at last an opportunity to use the courage she has needed as a survivor to face what has happened to her, in the open.

I think and I think, and my brain seems to grow bigger than my skull can continue to contain. My thought seems to throb with the pitiless vastness of this new knowledge, and with the knowledge of pain I have not even been able to guess at, beyond the walls of the room where we meet, out into the streets, streaming into the thoughts of women who hurry past. One in ten. At the very least, one in ten have been sexually abused by a trusted adult. One in ten struggles alone with the lost ability ever to trust again. But when we do find ourselves being asked to trust again in 'someone who knows', someone we conceive to be 'up there' in a professional capacity, there can come again that disbelief, accusation, indifference, scorn, that further abuse of power, which has been invested in the name of healing, and which only reaffirms our lack of worth in our own eyes.

[. . .]

It took me a long time to understand some of what was happening in the group. Often, I would go home feeling very torn-up inside. At times I felt a oneness with individual survivors which went so deep that I felt almost as if I was them, although in every exterior way we were different. Perhaps these were moments of love. There would also be enormous rage on the others' behalf. We all experienced this. After a time it came to me that this seemingly passive activity of listening and absorbing, and the responses of pain and anger for another person, were familiar. The 'other person' was me. I felt within me something of what I had felt happening when I looked at and absorbed the words I had written down in the letters about my childhood. Previously we had allowed ourselves to feel for each other. That was all right. But for each of us, sooner or later, came the awareness that the anguish we felt for each other was also, and with increasing intensity as the realisation dawned, for ourselves.

We had feared and fought against self-pity, fended off the indulgence of pain, but the hard accepting silence which had become a lifetime's habit was undermined by others' tears, tears of sorrow, rage, loneliness, meaninglessness, tears which each survivor had held inside, unable to release in any other way. For each of us had taught ourselves with consummate skill not to feel, not to cry, not to know about the great reservoir of grief within us. More than anything we had been afraid of losing the innermost grip on our control, of 'letting ourselves down', of being swept away in the deluge of our own tears. But owning what belonged to us, with support, brought some measure of control, and this increased as we explored the extent of our anguish, and discovered at last that it was finite, and that we had survived, and could now go on to live.

[. . .]

FIFTY-FIVE

EFFECTIVE TEAM MEETINGS

Sue Bailey

Working in a team has its advantages and disadvantages. The obvious good aspects that we would all acknowledge are the feelings of support, a joint purpose, and possibly a shared identity. For example, there is the comfort of being in a professional group – nurses or therapists or social workers – or perhaps working in the same geographical location to improve the situation of local people. We may work from the same base, for the same general practice or on the same unit, and what we have in common is our client group. Yet often the disadvantages of working in a team are concealed and less well articulated: they can often feel like failures. Meaningful, useful communication or the lack of it can be at the root of the problem.

We can take these perceived failures personally. The cry 'Communication is poor' is heard in every workplace and each of us may feel we have not communicated well. When this happens we may feel or be made to feel that we are not a 'team player', especially when we disagree with our colleagues or challenge a way of working, a belief or a practice.

'You haven't communicated with us' is a charge sometimes put to colleagues who are trying to effect a change or an improvement.

Team working is not about always agreeing with your colleagues or failing to challenge the perceived agreed position. It is, among other things, about good communication.

Teams work best when there is synergy, when the combined energies create something new. I once worked in a team where the regular team meeting, designed to effect regular communication, had a centrally driven agenda devised by the manager. Agenda items put forward by the team were relegated to 'any other business' or the team was told, through the secretary, that these items were not relevant. In short, it was not a team meeting as no real communication that the team was requesting could happen. It was not given a space in which to operate. The team meeting was a one-way exchange between the manager and the team. Challenges or new thinking were treated with hurt surprise. The effect of this denial of the team agenda and the guilt of having caused pain to the manager had a detrimental effect. To avoid the manager's disapproval, the team took their need to communicate underground. Gossip replaced debate. Tribes and schisms formed within the team as individuals aligned themselves with a particular way of thinking, a cause or a new idea that had no meaningful place in which to be debated. This team began not only thinking alike but also dressing alike. I found myself wearing clothes that were totally unsuited to my personality in order to fit in.

Team meetings were followed by one-to-one sessions where each person's behaviour within the team meeting was analysed. Any divergence from universal approval was criticised. The manager was looking for a team of look-alikes or sound-alikes. Her view of a team was a group of people who were like-minded and agreed all the time. Any diversion from this was seen as a threat to the overall well-being of the team.

How can we communicate in our teams without presenting such a difficult challenge that the team ceases to function while the internal rifts caused by challenge to the status quo are managed and resolved? Jay (1995) says that team meetings are vital to creating a sense of team spirit and that running effective meetings is a key management skill. My experience is, having suffered team meetings and team dynamics that impeded the functioning of the team, I knew that when I managed a team of people the meetings had to be different.

I asked my team what they wanted from their meetings with me and each other and what they resoundingly said was 'We need to communicate, not just listen to an agenda. We need to use the meeting to debate and discuss and work through our issues.' Consequently, I threw the agenda open, and the team drove the discussion. By managing the time allotted to each issue raised, we kept the meeting within the time we all thought was appropriate. We agreed some core agenda items that we knew would always come up or that needed constant attention: for example, projects that were in progress, staffing issues and customer feedback.

The meetings were scheduled at a time when other crucial meetings would not be happening, so loyalty was not divided, and at a location in the organisation where we could all park our cars, get some tea and coffee, and have a decent chair and a table to work at in a proper meeting room. I have lost count of the meetings I attended where none of these basic essentials were provided.

The end result was 100% attendance (apart from annual leave), enjoyment and engagement of all the team, outcomes in respect of targets hit and deadlines met, and the envy of colleagues in other teams who asked us how we did it.

REFERENCE

Jay, R. (1995) *Build a Great Team!*, London, Pitman/Institute of Management Foundation.

FIFTY-SIX

SHOWING THE WORKING: LEADERSHIP AND TEAM CULTURE

Janet Seden

Hindsight is a wonderful thing. Looking back and reflecting on team leaders and the teams I have been part of as a social worker brings back more positive experiences of communication and relationships than poor ones. Perhaps I have been very lucky. Although, looking back, I am very aware of choosing jobs on the basis of who the team manager was, knowing that in a stressful job such as the probation service or child and family social work, the way the team works together or not makes such a difference to individual workers. The job is stressful anyway so that knowing you can rely on a 'chat' or longer discussion with your colleagues or a supervisor who will listen and offer helpful advice makes all the difference between coping and not coping. It makes the workplace feel energising and creative rather than anxious and oppressive. I have experienced both climates but the learning always came from the people who could inspire by example.

As a young and very new probation officer, the first manager I had was someone who chose to work with a team composed of 50% new recruits and he specialised in developing the skills of officers in their first year. However, he always made sure half his team had substantial work experience. He was known for his patience, and being relaxed, good humoured and approachable, but he took his roles and responsibilities towards us very seriously, in the sense that he 'watched our backs' and let us know about it.

He would pop his head round the door in the morning and comment, 'I see Mrs X who you supervise is on the court list again.' Silence while

I thought, 'Oh no, I had forgotten I was supposed to check!' Someone else might have said, 'Have you checked the court list today?' Or been very critical and said, 'I see you forgot to check the list again.' Criticism would have frozen me into inertia – but his approach made it safe to say 'Sorry I didn't see – should I go down to court now?' And he would then advise either 'Yes, it's serious' or 'No, but be available', or 'No, go and do your visits, I'll cover'. I quickly learned to check the list properly myself, and to judge when to attend court urgently and when I could let the duty probation officer speak for me.

We all overheard the friendly comments and advice to others as he popped his head round the doors and quickly learned what was expected of the role. However, he wasn't Superman, and I will never forget him bellowing at an officer who did not get the message after several friendly reminders about the court list, 'Get to b. . ... court NOW!' Interestingly, no one complained, including the recipient of the abuse. I think we all recognised it as fair, if ill judged! Letting the service down in front of magistrates or judges by failing to be there when needed was serious, and this colleague was unfailingly and exasperatingly not there when you needed him.

Later, working in a busy social work team that took urgent calls from the public, I learned again the value of open teamwork. The team manager would sit with the two of us 'on duty' in the open plan office with his paperwork. As we took calls we could hear the advice the other worker was giving. There was also the expectation that if you were unsure how to respond you took the caller's name, address and number and found out what they were asking for. You then rang back after a few minutes of discussion with the team manager and the other worker. As the rota meant you worked with different colleagues and both team managers we all built up shared experience and expertise quickly. The discussions would be about what the service could or could not provide. The analysis of policy directives and resource availability – what should be offered, what should be said on the return call and what we had to respond to urgently by a home visit – was explored very carefully each time.

This daily learning in twos and threes fed into team discussions and the development of policy, so that the public was getting a quality and consistency of service that was constantly reviewed against agency policy and procedure. I also recall both these managers discussing with workers whether they felt 'safe' or 'competent' to make visits where clients had serious mental health issues or there were concerns for a child's safety. Where workers were genuinely unsure, the manager would either take the calls while both workers went out to visit the service user or go along too and perhaps wait outside.

The climate of trust in these teams was high between managers and staff, and very popular with students from local universities seeking their practice placements.

Another team I worked in took long-term and complex children and families support work, where there were serious concerns about the children's welfare. We were in offices in twos and threes and, in my little group, we had really difficult work supporting families who were often close to their children being taken into care. We would spend the first 20 minutes of most mornings drinking coffee and talking about work with each other, sharing ideas and concerns and often solutions or sources of financial or other help for families. We also laughed a lot and this really helped deal with the stress. The team manager took a relaxed attitude to the amount of coffee drinking and peer chat in the team room, recognising that it was 'problem-solving' and work activity. This was a team where we looked forward to meeting and sharing and it felt safe to share work anxieties and to ask for help if personal circumstances made it necessary.

In fact the team culture saved the manager a lot of work because certainly the three people in my office provided peer supervision and back-up for each other informally, building a set of relationships with each other. It meant often if you were late or ill the others had 'covered' your work by taking calls. Because we knew how each other worked this seldom caused problems. If someone was off sick for a few days or on holiday there was little need for formal reallocation of work: those who knew it would stand in for the short term. These relationships were usually reciprocal and no one took advantage of other people's willingness to help out. This meant we usually went to formal supervision with ideas and plans for work, which the manager could then discuss, and either approve or ask us to change. Most service users would know more than one worker if they were a family where crises happened often and responses were needed urgently. The team leader would also make formal opportunities at team meetings for us to present work issues for discussion in turns. This too was very useful information sharing and learning.

The team manager worked late most days, usually being the last person to go home. This meant if you paid a visit at 4.30 pm when children were in from school and had concerns, she would usually be there for consultation as needed afterwards. We worked as a team responding to the neighbourhood, and saw the work as a team responsibility, not just that of the key worker. So if, for example, suddenly several children in one family had to be moved to foster placement in an emergency, we all dropped less urgent work and helped, either with form filling, transport, or settling a child or reassuring a parent. This sounds 'cosy' and, looking back, it was special, but it was a robust and supportive system. It stands out as good experience of a team working together to support families, and the team had a reputation for being a good place to work.

Many of the child care and other social work teams in local authorities work well because of a sharing of pressures and an atmosphere where worries and uncertainties can be honestly voiced. Sometimes, though, it was not so good because there was an 'If you can't stand the heat get out of the kitchen' approach from a manager. Such teams would have the highest staff turnover and be less pleasant to work in. Sometimes, however, the relationships and dynamics of a team went wrong. In one team this happened when a new person joined. Everyone helped the new person to settle in as usual. There is a high staff turnover on child care teams and we often had part-time help, students and social work assistants coming and going, but being part of the work while they were with us. All seemed fine until the new person introduced her own personal difficulties into the informal discussions, talking at length about herself. We then began to notice that she was spending up to an hour in one colleague's office fairly regularly being 'helped' and when we asked we were told that she had asked the colleague to keep it 'confidential'. This colleague was someone we all respected and so we thought, well, a bit of extra support to settle in and handle the work seemed all right. It was accepted that the rest of us supported students and new workers from time to time.

However, after a while, the first colleague had to say she could not spend so much time listening to the new person's difficulties. The new colleague then started 'visiting' another colleague, until she also felt it was not OK – but again it had been 'confidential'. Eventually, one by one, we all seemed to be 'sucked in' and the whole office was listening to and supporting one person. We were all sympathetic – the job was tough and stressful – but the more we listened and responded, the more time seemed to be spent, until it felt like the whole team was preoccupied with one person. Also the 'confidential' bit had been a mistake – in the past all office conversations had been open to everyone. This was a new ball game – and we did not want to play. Nobody knew who knew what and the atmosphere was getting uncomfortable.

So we individually withdrew, from the new colleague and each other, basically because the children and families we worked with had to come first. At this point the team manager understandably, seeing the new person as 'isolated', started to extend the new colleague's supervision sessions and to stay late to support her at work. The outcome was we were all formally asked to share the workload and offer support in a team meeting. This did not go down too well as everyone was stretched, and we had already offered loads of support, apparently unnoticed and unrecognised. The atmosphere got worse and what had been a good system of informal networking failed. People got irritated because their supervision was cancelled. The boundaries on short breaks for informal chat, which we all observed, had been broken and colleague-to-colleague support had become therapy for one person. This was fairly sustainable until the, by now, not-so-new colleague began criticising team members for 'not helping' her and 'marginalising' her, relaying this to the team manager, who had to take her allegations seriously.

This consumed more supervision time and created havoc in the team. Individually we started staying out on visits and stopped going to team meetings, which were tense with everyone feeling uncomfortable but no one being willing to be the first to air the difficulties. One person got another job on another team. No one felt they could share the small personal pieces of news that we used to just support each other, for fear of it becoming a problem or too much, as it had with the new worker.

Eventually the person was off sick and relocated to another team but everyone felt guilty. The team culture became more formal. (Was that better? It didn't feel better). The trust and spontaneity were lost and the meeting of each other's needs in a supportive reciprocal way had gone. Also, in trying to keep the balance between professional work and personal support, each one of us was accused of undermining someone else who wanted more than any of us had time to give. When the team manager offered intensive support that also failed. The team manager worked very hard with each individual's issues and a transparent workload system after that to get the team back together. Culture when it works can be fragile and I learned something valuable about personal/professional boundaries through that experience.

Another team leader of a similar team modelled practice in a helpful way. Her office door was always open in the mornings from 8.30 to 10.00 when the most urgent issues would be coming to the team's attention. If we did not call on her, she would just check that she was not missing anything where her advice was needed before she went off to management meetings or other tasks. She would build relationships with the team by organising to be with us all for lunch on team meeting day – and be visible in the staff room for lunch breaks on other days, thus giving us permission to do the same.

This same team manager, however, was very good at saying, 'I wouldn't do that like that because . . .' and 'If you do X you will find that . . .', or sharing her own experience: 'You know I did it that way once and it went terribly wrong because . . .' We all respected this openness, especially as it extended to accompanying us on home visits where difficult things might have to be said and she would leave you to talk, only coming in if you felt stuck. I can still picture her in clients' homes giving encouraging smiles and nods when what I was saying was helpful or chipping in where I missed something. It was always possible to ask for support when sensitive visits about issues of abuse or neglect were needed.

All the team felt confident about the support she offered. In team meetings and individually within the team she would be clear about what she thought was good or poor practice and why, but she unfailingly took responsibility with senior management for the team's work and actions and, whatever was said to the team, we were defended to senior management. In an environment where fine judgements are made and courses of action are difficult to assess and get right, this kind of team leadership was greatly valued. She was also, like the team leader of the other team, absolutely and passionately on the service user's side – an attitude which was both infectious and unstoppable.

In hindsight these team leaders offered honesty, respect and genuineness to their teams and could convey it through words and actions. They all used styles of relating which were friendly but formal and all stuck to the rules, procedures and values of the agency and expected of us, but somehow without getting stuck in management speak or jargon. For me a good team leader:

- communicates what you are expected to do, but chooses words that do not criticise or belittle, especially when your practice is less than desirable
- is honest about your failings and offers a way to do better
- offers encouragement and recognition for what is going well
- builds relationships that are open and engages at the human level of team interaction (e.g. lunch, coffee breaks) without being intrusive
- leads by example – you can watch and hear ways of doing and speaking that are good practice
- leaves space for the team members to build relationships with and support each other
- retains a sense of humour and proportion while still keeping to the work tasks
- conveys respect, genuineness and empathy to staff within the boundaries of the work relationship
- makes opportunities for team members to learn together and from each other.

FIFTY-SEVEN

WORKING WITH TEAMS

Peter Miles

As a training consultant, I have worked with a wide variety of teams in small and large businesses, universities and schools. I have also worked with teams in the NHS and in other social care and health settings including charities and voluntary organisations. More recently, I have experienced health and social care teams at work from a user perspective both as a client and as my parents and in-laws become more regular users of both institutional and home care.

As an inveterate team 'watcher', I have learned two key things. Firstly, there are many different ways of observing and thinking about teams – different perspectives give different insights. Secondly, teams are difficult to predict. This means analysing teams and team dynamics is problematic. In this article, I reflect on what I have learned about teams with particular reference to communications within teams and between teams.

When it comes to teams, does size matter? It does because it is very hard to have the same feelings, either as a team member or as a disinterested observer, about a small, tight-knit team and about a large, perhaps physically distributed, team. Larger teams are different from small teams. They need different processes and different ways of communicating. A junior staff member in a well known London hospital once said to me, 'I don't know how it is done but I feel both part of this ward team and a member of the much bigger directorate team.' I was not absolutely sure how it was done either. However, in that directorate team of 200 staff, they did spend time ensuring everybody understood and was committed to the quality of care they aimed to provide their patients. They also put much effort into communicating how much individual and team contributions were valued. So both sense of purpose and belonging seem important to teams, whatever their size.

In any team, it is usually possible to identify both formal and informal communications processes. For example, I recently worked with several research teams in a national health charity. Two of these teams interested me especially. When I talked to members of each team, they claimed communication generally worked very well. The teams were of a similar size, had been in existence about the same amount of time, were made up of people with similar backgrounds, had similar demanding research targets, and had very similar laboratory and office accommodation.

In one team (Team A), most communication was very formal. There were regular meetings of the whole team and of key sub-teams, minutes of all meetings were taken and issued, all team members had access to an electronic message board, team members had job descriptions and formal performance management targets, and research and reporting protocols were contained in a manual which was prominently on display in all work settings.

Team B, in contrast, avoided meetings, recorded very little in writing, largely ignored many of the formal procedures that the research division and the parent organisation laid down, and seemed to rely on a network of informal communications between members and sub-groups. Team members were aware that they relied largely on informal contact. They told me this meant they made a point of meeting for coffee, having lunch together from time to time, chatting at the water cooler, and leaving each other 'Post-its'.

As I got to know Team B better, I discovered that they also used email to communicate extensively with each other. It had become custom and practice to copy all colleagues into nearly all emails that passed between team members. Key emails sent to or received from other people in the rest of the organisation were also forwarded to all team members. So Team B members could make choices about how well informed they were. They could choose to read or not to read their emails.

By contrast, in Team A, the main form of communication was the meetings which all members were expected to attend. They could miss a meeting only if they had a very good excuse, i.e. too busy or very senior! I attended one of Team A's meetings. It was a formal affair with a written agenda, minutes were read and approved, and each item on the agenda had a time attached to it. The chair closed any discussion when the minute taker indicated time was up. Not that there was much discussion because the chair, the formal leader of the team, did most of the talking.

I find being a fly on the wall at team meetings interesting because they often seem to be microcosms of how communications work in a team more generally. At some team meetings, the predominant mode of communication is one person talks, mostly the formal leader, and the remainder of the team listens. In this type of briefing meeting, at times the team leader is communicating with every member of the team and at other times is effectively just talking to one person in the team. The other team members then have a choice. They either listen or they switch off: they disengage.

By contrast, in some ward and unit meetings, most of the communication is between the team members. In this type of team, communication is multi-channelled and engages everyone. I have observed this kind of communication in both inter-agency and multidisciplinary teams. In one inter-agency team, it was quite hard to spot the formal leader. Leadership seemed to shift round the team depending on the nature and the demands of the task. In contrast, in a multidisciplinary team, it was very clear who the formal leader was. The senior medic took a leadership role but she was not the focus of all communication. Her function was to facilitate the multi-channel communication in this well-established team.

Many health and social care staff experience a fluid pattern of team working. They move between different types of team apparently seamlessly, for example from a team of peer professionals, to a multidisciplinary team, to an inter-agency team. Many teams have sub-teams or are a sub-team of a yet larger team. For example, a shift team may consist of staff who all belong to the same bigger, permanent team. Many hospital wards have this kind of team. However, in social care I have worked with shift teams whose members each came from different, larger teams, for example nurses, social workers and clerical staff.

What Teams A and B, the inter-agency team and the multidisciplinary team, have in common is that they are, to all intents and purposes, permanent teams. Membership may change but the team tasks are long-term. Many people spend their day-to-day work in teams such as these. However, much work in many organisations is project-based. Project teams are temporary teams with a planned life span and usually consist of staff from other teams. Their members may be seconded full-time to the project team or they may come to the project part-time. A different type of temporary team is the one that comes together occasionally, for example a disaster response team. Its members leave their permanent team, work intensely alongside colleagues from other permanent teams, then return to their 'home' team.

Within this wide variety of type and structure, teams also appear to have their own life cycles. There are young teams, developing teams, adapting teams, mature teams, declining and dying teams. Next I want to focus on some of the issues that concern a team in the early stages of its formation. These are different from the issues that concern a team in the later stages of its life.

Early on in its formation, a team needs to spend time and energy on these sorts of questions. Are all team members clear about the task and what we are trying to achieve? Do we have the right skill mix? Do we share values, expectations, aspirations, hopes and fears? How will we be led? How will we communicate with each other? Can we trust and support one another? Often, at this stage, it is important to answer the question 'Who is a member of the team?' So, in this unit or clinic, who is in the team and who is not? Over the last 20 years, I have seen a significant change in ideas about team membership not just in hospitals, GP surgeries and other health and social care settings but also, for example, in schools.

The model of the team just consisting of so-called professionals is largely gone. Only nurses, or only nurses and doctors, or only qualified teachers or social workers are in the team. Who is in the team is now much more likely to be determined in relation to the service user. All those who provide services of whatever kind to users are members of the team. Administrative staff, ancillary and cleaning staff are included. This change has been much influenced by studies of team working by researchers such as Meredith Belbin (1995) who argue that a team is a collection of differences and not of similarities. It seems an effective team needs a diversity of skills, functions and roles.

This diversity is often provided by other staff who join the team from time to time but are not based in a ward, clinic or care home and, indeed, are members of several other teams as well. Teams often consist of both core personnel and others who join and leave the team depending on the needs of the task and/or client. This way of working brings challenges to both the core team members and those on the periphery, not least about how communications function. Issues of competing agendas and loyalties also have to be dealt with in these sorts of teams.

I experienced this preoccupation with core and periphery in a care home for adults with learning difficulties where I did some voluntary work. In this home, there was a great deal of ambiguity about who was in the team and who was not. The rhetoric of the home was that all staff, the residents, the representatives of the funders and the many volunteers were involved in both day-to-day and longer-term decisions about the running of the home. The home manager talked a lot about the need for all these groups to work as a team and often spoke at meetings about the need for good team work and about social and other events in the home as team-building activities. However, in practice I was only an insider sometimes. It became evident that the manager, his deputy and one of the funders took all key decisions. In many organisations, there is much rhetoric about teams and team working. As in so many other situations, when it comes to teams, rhetoric and reality are often not the same.

Ideas about who is inside and who is outside are important because they help define a team's boundaries. Other factors add to this definition, for example the physical space a team occupies, the team's location in relation to its clients and to other teams, the training members receive, the language a team uses, how team members dress, and even how breaks and other off-duty times are spent. A team's boundaries give a sense of belonging to its members and provide protection, a shelter to return to for sustenance and support. This is especially important for team members who work with clients in tough settings. I have experienced teams who provide superb support to staff working with dying patients, seriously ill children, and mentally ill clients. On the other hand, I have seen health and social care staff with very challenging roles who seem to get little or no support, both practical and emotional, from their team.

However, boundaries can also be barriers. They can keep out new members, ideas, resources, and awkward questions about a team's purpose. Teams can become isolated, out-of-touch, self-serving and preoccupied with meeting the needs of their members. This can happen to teams that have been in existence for some time, to teams that have been very successful, and to teams facing great odds. The inquiries into child protection tragedies have shown how boundaries between teams, for example between those in different agencies, can lead to a breakdown in communications and the need for what has been called 'open teamwork' (Payne, 2000). Boundaries might provide a safe container but they also need to be worked through and across.

As well as managing its boundaries, a challenge to a well-established team can be significant changes of team personnel. Some of the original members may have left the team or be about to depart. These may be the members who somehow embody the goals, values, aspirations and unspoken rules of the team. Their leaving is a significant loss to other team members but may also be an opportunity to revitalise the team. The team may need to revisit questions about its purpose, structure and ways of working. I have helped a variety of teams in health and social care ask and get answers to key questions such as 'How do others see us?' Are the clients we provide services to getting what they want? What about those who provide us with services and resources? How do they see us? How are communications working in this team and between this team and other groups?

It is possible to find teams whose complete membership changes but the team continues. Such teams may have been established and had their tasks and purposes defined by the wider organisation. So, rather than the members embodying the team, how team members behave is enshrined in systems, protocols and procedures. Team members know how to act and interact because they have received thorough training and understand each other's roles. The most obvious example of this kind of team is a hospital resuscitation team who respond to emergency 'crash' calls. Procedures, protocols, routines, roles, etc. are clearly laid down so that the team can function whichever members are present. Likewise, an eye clinic I attended never seemed to have many of the same administrative, nursing or medical staff present but the processing of patients appeared to be well orchestrated. Perhaps I could not see what went on behind the scenes.

In a well-established, highly effective team, communication can be virtually wordless: a look or a small gesture can be a complex message. Alternatively, team members may have developed a shorthand way of talking that outsiders may find difficult to follow. Teams that have trained intensively together, gone through difficult times together, or overcome great odds often show these characteristics. They are comparatively easy to spot, for instance in a two-person ambulance crew or in a surgical team in an operating theatre. The intensity of the task in hand demands a high level of trust and mutual understanding. I have also found this type of communication in other settings, for example in long-term care teams, where the pressures are less intense but where what is not said is as important as what is said.

It is an interesting paradox that what can indicate a highly effective team may also be a sign that a team is in some way dysfunctional. The things a team cannot talk about speak volumes about the state of the team. An established team often has all sorts of not-talked-about assumptions about the team and its members. For example, a physio-therapist working with children who have learning and behavioural difficulties said to me, 'In this team I can't really talk about what I find difficult to cope with because round here not being able to cope is a sign of weakness.' A midwife, who regularly worked more than her official hours, reported, 'I don't like to take back time owing to me because the team expectation is that we are around to support each other at all times, particularly at the shift handover. I can't walk out on a woman in labour or let my colleagues down.'

Language is a way of exercising power both within and by a team. Listen to the ways teams talk with each other both in formal settings and informally, for example at break time or even in other social contexts. Listen to the stories they tell about their clients, their successes and their difficulties. Listen to the language that is used. What are the themes? What is the dominant discourse? How is power mediated and exercised?

A team that develops its own way of talking can also operate in ways that exclude. A few years ago I lay in a strange bed, eyes bandaged and in some pain and a team of nurses and doctors discussed 'my case' in a language that I had no access to. At the time, I and my family reacted with both distress and anger. In hindsight, I see that I felt excluded by the team and now I ask the question 'Shouldn't patients, and their families, be active members of their care team?'

Some of the ways of thinking about teams I have reflected on here are in some senses limited in that they assume that teams are largely fixed identities, with for example defined and definable boundaries and identifiable life cycles. However, teams in reality are ever-changing, shifting, hard-to-pin-down entities which have both declared and undeclared purposes. They have permeable boundaries, they change shape and size, and they grow and change in an organic way. They are also places in which both conscious and unconscious motivations and behaviours of team members are played out. People who are members of several teams probably experience them differently and can move between the teams, mediating their identity as required and choosing what kind of team member to be.

In conclusion, I recently watched and listened to a group of staff who were caring for my 89-year-old father. (Well, the truth is I was eavesdropping on them.) There was a lot of tension in the team and two of the members were arguing fiercely. Their body language indicated defensiveness, separateness and division. When they stopped debating their own circumstances, the gist of what they then said was 'at least in this team we are better than the other teams in this unit'. I drove home worried about the quality of care my father was receiving. Later I was surprised to learn that, from his perspective, this team 'were the best' he had ever experienced and they really 'delivered the goods'.

So I learned yet again what of course I already knew in my role as a so-called objective team watcher. Whatever way you analyse teams, from whatever perspective and on whatever level, your own values and beliefs will be present. The people in organisations who lead teams and advocate teamwork claim much for the benefits of teams and teamworking. We can challenge their claims critically from knowledge of our own beliefs and values about teams. I have learned from the people I have worked with that they desire both to be members of a team and to hold on to their own individual identity. This sets up conflicts and tensions. When I am in need of health and social services, I want to be part of the team assigned to my care but I also want to keep my separate identity. I can just about work with this paradox. Can you?

REFERENCES

Belbin, M. (1995) *Team Roles at Work*, London, Butterworth-Heinemann.
Payne, M. (2000) *Teamwork in Multiprofessional Care*, Basingstoke, Palgrave.

FIFTY-EIGHT

'REMIND ME WHO I AM, AGAIN' – EXTRACT 2

Linda Grant

My mother adores hospitals after a first unfortunate visit when she went in as a child to have her tonsils removed and cried because it was the Passover and nobody brought her the prescribed unleavened bread. There were two visits to the Oxford Maternity Hospital in Liverpool at which, with her dead to the world, her daughters were surgically removed from her abdomen. When she came home with her second bundle of joy she brought with her a half-completed jumper suit in black wool flecked with silver which she had begun to knit but abandoned because she couldn't be bothered. It knocked around the house for years, ending up as dusters. I bet it's still somewhere in the world, indestructible though incomplete.

At Poole Hospital, this time, things aren't quite the same. The GP says he is not convinced that she has had a heart attack at all. Michele thinks he sees the dramatic episode with the after-hours call and the ambulance and the rushed admission as another form of attention-seeking. She's always coming in to the surgery, he complains. I go to see him. He is a vain, shallow, good-looking man with a case-load which he feels to be heavily burdened by geriatric patients though if he had wanted to avoid them he should not have taken up practice in Bournemouth. None the less, he finds my mother particularly difficult. She thinks she has a hold on him, for when she contracted cancer he had wanted to put her straight into hospital for a mastectomy – an old woman like her, what did she need with two breasts or even any? But Michele manipulates the system to get her taken on as a temporary patient by her own doctor, which opens the door

Source: Grant, L. *Remind Me Who I am, Again.* London: Granta Publications, 1998.
Reproduced by permission.

to second opinion at Barts, and so she was saved from that grisly fate. Now she thinks that gives her the right to demand his attention at will. She has told me this herself.

I ask him about her memory. 'Old people forget things,' he says, dismissively. 'My own mother forgets things.'

So for the first week after she comes out of hospital I stay with her as she is still too weak to care for herself and though the hospital had suggested a few days in a nursing home, she has turned them down flat. 'Why do I need to go there,' she demands, 'when I have daughters to look after me?' I am told that she mustn't do any heavy cleaning, like hoovering or moving furniture. I ring Dorset Social Services and ask if she could be assigned a home help. The Welfare State exists only to a minimal extent in Bournemouth, I discover, with its Tory council and huge population of elderly residents. With £9,000 invested in a unit trust and the ownership of her own home, my mother does not qualify for state assistance. I am given a list of private agencies but no recommendation. I select one at random.

The owner comes to the house. She wears high boots and perches on the edge of my mother's gilded chairs, nodding furiously. She seems pleasant and sympathetic. My mother likes her and Ms Big Boots thinks she has just the woman to suit. I think so too, when I meet her, for she is Liverpool Black, one of that odd ethnic minority which did not come to Britain as immigrants from the Caribbean in the 1950s and 1960s but is descended from black American and African seamen who married or fathered children on the girls they met on shore leave. She had nursed her own mother in her own home until her death. The first thing she does is bring her husband over to fit a hand-rail into the tiled wall beside the bath. We think we have struck lucky.

'I'm determined I'm going to make a friend of her,' my mother says, 'so I can keep her.'

The bill is sent to my sister and me.

For two or three days my mother seems to be rallying fast, speaking of short coach trips to the surrounding countryside and taking up her old work holding the hands of her 'dears' at the day centre. I meet the neighbours who are in and out with cakes and biscuits and cold fried fish. Her friends from the League throng the house. Offers of kosher meals on wheels are made. She can come back to her old volunteer role as soon as she is well, her place will always be held for her.

I go out for a long walk along the front in the autumn sunshine, kicking sand amongst the dunes, watch the late holidaymakers on the beach and locals brewing tea in their beach huts. Here is the Cumberland Hotel where I had my first-ever cigarette and went green and was sick; where I kissed a boy on the avenues that are lined with pine trees, and I wonder what has become of him – a dad now, probably, with daughters of his own. I think of my father's oscillating path between flat, bookmakers, pub and promenade in the brief time he had had there, the incongruity of a pensioner's bus pass in his black pocket instead of the jangling keys to his Humber Hawk with its cream leather interior. When they first came my mother sat on the beach and closing her eyes, raised her face to the sun.

'It bores me,' she says, when I ask her why she doesn't do that any more.

When I get back the doctor's locum is there. The minute I'd gone she had felt pains in her chest. The locum gives her a spray to hiss into the roof of her mouth. 'You've had an angina attack but if you use this spray whenever you feel it coming on, the pain will pass,' she said. It's a shame I don't look at the clock because it would have told me the precise time she became an invalid.

She will not eat the meals on wheels. 'Horrible.' She will not go back to the League. 'I'm not ready.' She does not want to see visitors. 'I can't be bothered with them.'

I send off for brochures for sheltered housing thinking that this might be a solution to her problems. She looks at them and rejects them. 'Too far out,' she says. 'No shops. Here I've got everything on my doorstep.' She's quite right. Those places are designed for people who like a garden, who want to be just a hop away from fields and hills and rivers, and those pleasures bore her stiff, or rather she likes nature in the same way that I do: it's scenery, exterior décor for the motorway.

During that week I injure my back helping her into the bath. I had had back trouble for years but I am to notice increasingly that the bouts recur every time I visit my mother. The physiotherapist says it's stress. It *is* stressful, swallowing down my irritation at what I see as her malingering and her bored repetitions, due, I believe, to her not having much to talk about.

A few months later she tells me, 'I've sacked the home help, you know. She was useless.'

'I don't see how you can sack her,' I say, 'since it's Michele and I who are paying for her.' The agency finds someone else.

My mother also mentions that the hospital has diagnosed mild diabetes. Her own mother had had the same thing. It is to be controlled by diet. After a lifetime's consumption of sweets, cakes and biscuits she is now forbidden all sugar.

Diabetes is one of the many factors that increases the amount of arteriosclerosis in blood vessels. Most diabetics, if they have badly controlled diabetes, are more likely to get heart attacks, strokes, blood-vessel damage in the eye, which is one of the reasons they're more likely to go blind. They are more likely to have problems with their legs, which eventually lead to amputation. Diabetes aggravates or causes arteriosclerosis. And that is true of late-onset diabetes, to a lesser extent than early-onset but it is still a risk factor. Diabetes is an early-warning symptom of Multi-Infarct Dementia (MID). I often wonder if a sweet tooth cost my mother her mind and if it will cost me mine.

27 April 1993

Dear Doctor _____

I wonder if you would consider seeing Rose Grant and taking over her care. _____, an old friend, recommended you as the person best able to deal with this problem. In brief she is a dementing lady with two distantly located daughters. I was asked to give an opinion by a mutual third party. I enclose correspondence from her daughter Linda.

Mrs. Rose Grant and her husband retired to Bournemouth but unfortunately he died two years later leaving her somewhat isolated. As Linda says, her mother is rather resentful that they do not live in an extended family environment in Liverpool. Medically she has a history of diabetes (mainly diet-controlled), ischaemic heart disease, and carcinoma of the breast. She may have had a cardiac infarct eighteen months ago and went to Oxford for further tests. She certainly seems to suffer from angina but I suspect some of her pain is muscular-skeletal and in part related to her lymphoedema following axillary node dissection. Her medication includes Nitro, Isosorbide, Tenormin 100 mg a day, Diltiazem 60 mg t.d.s., Aspirin 75 mg a day, Prednisolone 5 mg (?why), Zantac 150 mg b.d., and Gaviscon prescribed since the infarct.

The major problem is of short-term memory loss. This predated her cardiac trouble by two or three years but has been worse since then. The family report a stepwise deterioration consistent with vascular disease. The patient herself retains insight into the difficulty. Self-care seems to be reasonable and continence is preserved. She is still able to go out of the house and does not feel lost. She claims to feel depressed – her sleep is normal but she is occasionally tearful. She has a home help but I suspect she does not do much cooking.

On examination she is reasonably well orientated and scores 24/34 in an extended MTS. I did not find her overtly clinically depressed. The pulse was 80 suggesting she may not be using the Beta blocker. The blood pressure was 150/90. There was no cardiac failure and no abnormal signs in the chest or abdomen. In the central nervous system the fundi were normal but I thought there was a slight weakness of the right arm and leg with increased reflexes.

There is lymphoedema of the left arm. Overall I feel she has a dementing illness almost certainly on the basis of vascular disease. I am not sure how many clinics she is attending but feel she needs to be under a single umbrella. Whether all the medication is necessary (and indeed if she is taking it) is uncertain. The Beta blocker may be contributing to her mental state. She may benefit from an anti-depressant. I feel she requires a district nurse to advise on medication and to provide a daily drug dispenser, and to monitor her dietary type and intake. She may require a health visitor or a CPN to monitor her functional state. I wonder if you would kindly consider taking her on and seeing her. I am sure in the first instance the family would be happy for you to see her on a private basis although in the long term NHS care would be more appropriate as they are not insured. Thank you very much for your help.

With best wishes,
Yours sincerely

Cc GP
Linda Grant

This is the time when people say to me, 'How's your mum?' and I reply, 'For God's sake, don't ask.' The time of the Hundred Years War when it's more the depression than the memory loss that I notice. 'I'm so depressed, I'm so depressed. Can't anyone take it away?' The slammed phones. The aborted visits. People with Alzheimer's often do not know what their own condition is. One of MID's cruellest tricks is to preserve in its victim until quite a late stage, some insight into what is going on in their mind, so they can observe themselves lose their own sanity. Depression and emotional instability is a marked characteristic of this disease and who wouldn't be miserable, watching themselves going mad.

So Michele and I have consulted our friends in the caring professions and the address of a Harley Street specialist has been given, the expedition to Harley Street organised – only the best for our mother and now we know what's the matter.

Sixty pounds has been well spent there. He has written to a colleague in Bournemouth assessing her health, suggesting that she be assigned to his care. [. . .]

On the tube, after the appointment, I say to my mother, 'It isn't Alzheimer's, you know. It's something called Multi-Infarct Dementia, little strokes. But not Alzheimer's.'

She replies, 'Thank God you told me. Because that's what I've been so worried about.'

A moment later she asks: 'Did the consultant say what was wrong with me?'

I have suggested to him that he try to talk her into going into sheltered housing. 'I think it may be a bit late for that,' he replies.

At any rate, *we* now know that *she* knows. Michele later believed that this was why she had dropped her friends, couldn't be bothered, never went out, didn't return their calls. That she was perfectly well aware of what was happening to her and was ashamed, embarrassed and afraid of their response. She had cut herself off because she could no longer manage the skills she needed to be in company. It was a proud, brave thing to do, though of course counter-productive. 'I cringe inside when someone tells me I'm repeating myself,' she had said once, in a rare acknowledgement to others of what was happening to her, so that just for that moment she was not covering up, putting on an act. For a lifetime of keeping up appearances had only prepared her for her greatest role, dementia, in which she did everything she could to pretend to the world that she was right as rain and could not stop to talk if she saw someone in the street for really, she had to dash, she was meeting a friend for morning coffee. Her neighbours told me that, later.

FIFTY-NINE

GHOSTS IN THE MACHINE: THE HIGHS AND LOWS OF MULTI-PROFESSIONAL AND INTER-AGENCY COMMUNICATION IN A MENTAL HEALTH SETTING

Charis Alland

I'm on an acute ward on constant observation. I'm desperate to leave – to be free to choose whether I live or die. I'm watching and waiting. Two of the three on night shift come into the day room. None of the staff speak to each other but my observer assumes one of them is there to relieve her. She leaves. Unsure which of them is with me I move out of the room to see who follows. For the first time in a month I'm alone in the corridor. I wait, afraid I'm mistaken, before following through what I've rehearsed in my head so long. Upstairs in a quiet corner of the dormitory a window opens onto the fire escape and my freedom. The opening of all the windows is limited but my weight loss serves me well. I squeeze through only to find myself caught on a nail. I can't move in or out and stay there for the next 45 minutes before, to my shame, I'm discovered.

Two weeks later I'm given my own CPA [Care Plan Assessment] paper-work to sign. I've had no involvement in its preparation. I'm distressed to see what's written: 'She has taken every opportunity to evade level 1 obser-vation.' I request that it is changed to reflect that I have only taken advant-age of the 'lapse' in observation. The request is denied. I don't sign.

Nine months later I'm settling into my room in a community residential house. I'm leaning out of the open window watching a magnificent sunset in a rare moment of peace. There's a thunder of footsteps up the stairs and vigorous banging on the door. One of the support workers tells me that I have to be moved to a room downstairs. I voice my distress. I'm settled and I like the room. I ask why but am given no answers. After hours of pleading I'm allowed to stay but a workman is called, out of hours, to nail up the window. I'm told it's not personal but policy. None of the other windows seem to be locked. After persistent questioning the manager admits that my records show a history of jumping out of windows. I try to explain the context of the incident, to say it's irrelevant now I'm free to walk out of a door. I fail to convince. Finally it takes my Consultant to reassure her. The window remains nailed up.

Two years on I ask to see a risk assessment that's part of a referral for another placement. I'm distressed to see noted that my suicidal ideation involves 'jumping from windows'. Finally I have the relationship with staff I need to rectify the long-standing misunderstanding. The record is amended.

For receivers of mental health services effective communication is an essential vehicle in the journey to recovery. The above account provides only a glimpse into the misunderstandings that can arise over time and across sectors and professions. Although it's perhaps inevitable that information is sometimes diluted, exaggerated or taken out of context, vigilance for such errors seems essential. For three and a half years my journey has taken me through the terrain of a private psychiatric hospital to the less privileged doors of an NHS hospital, a residential care setting, and community care, as well as through a transfer to a team in another part of the country. Being on an enhanced CPA, with a complex care plan, the people involved in my care have been many and varied and so with it the possibilities for misunderstanding. As the only constants on the journey we are, as service receivers, perhaps the ones most able to see when communication breaks down and are definitely the most exposed to the resulting chaos. Yet there is a danger that we are also the least heard or last to be involved in discussions, particularly when this happens.

There are many reasons why problems arise, from overworked and understaffed teams, to human fallibility, differing perspectives and professional rivalry. A blame culture adds to the need for some individuals to become defensive rather than accept responsibility when problems occur – so resolving them is consequently more difficult. The danger of scapegoating the receiver, particularly given that mental health issues often manifest in communication difficulties, is great. Often I had said to (or about) me: 'you didn't listen to what I said'; 'you didn't tell me that'; 'she misheard me/is playing up'; rather than: 'I didn't hear'; 'Perhaps I didn't explain it very well'; 'I'm sorry if I misunderstood/didn't pass that on/ that you felt misheard'; 'I wasn't given that information'.

Channels of communication are often more easily managed within homogenous groups or between smaller teams. When more than one system or profession is involved the diversity brings its own complications, with more scope for errors. The clearest example of this, on a corporate scale, came with my transition from a private hospital to the public sector. It was policy within the private hospital for records to remain confidential to the hospital. The community team taking over my care received limited information about the seven months I'd spent there (at NHS expense due to shortage of beds elsewhere). They didn't have the well-established links they might have had with their local NHS wards. The resulting lack of insight into my needs, together with a considerably less-resourced service, led to a breakdown in my care and a re-admission. At the time I interpreted the loss of support personally, felt undeserving, that my distress was being minimalised and my needs not taken seriously. It is only in hindsight it becomes clear how it was more to do with the service limitations and the problems liaising across the great divide that exists between the two sectors. It was, perhaps, easier for the NHS team to defend money-led decisions by reinterpreting and downsizing need according to what was available than to acknowledge the viewpoints of those previously involved in my care, and have to admit inferiority when they weren't able to provide what was necessary.

Maybe, more surprisingly, some of the problems that arose were in situations where there were no obvious differences or distances between those communicating. Sometimes more effort is given when it's assumed more explanation is required or it's acknowledged there's difference. Assumptions that others share your understanding or, because they are physically present, have heard what's being said can be the hidden cancer in communication. A common understanding of the context and use of language is also vital if there is to be consistency in approach; yet its existence may be taken for granted. For example, it could have been assumed that staff on the ward accepted and understood the same concept of constant observation. However the many different attitudes of the various individuals that became my observers showed this was far from the case. Some saw it as a pointless attention-giving exercise for troublesome individuals; some as merely custodial; some as a punishment and some as an opportunity for intensive therapy. Some were completely unaware why I, in particular, was being watched at all – one nurse sat fearfully watching me only to admit days later that she thought I was violent. It seemed these differences were never highlighted or questioned.

Another example is the issue of confidentiality. It may be assumed that the importance of this needs stressing to students, agency, or unqualified staff. Yet the lack of discretion came from qualified and senior staff often holding audible conversations about patients in corridors! (This also brings up the issue of the more practical barriers – of finding time and space to communicate effectively and ethically.)

From my experience it was obvious that the less autonomous, more hands on and less resourced the staff the greater the potential for miscommunication. In such environments morale and motivation can be low and the fear, frustration and anger tangible. In the close quarters of an acute ward it's often forgotten that patients aren't the only people being observed! Grievances soon become obvious. I often witnessed staff frustration unfairly taken out on 'difficult patients', so limiting the possibility for more helpful interactions. The information subsequently passed on to other professionals is inevitably coloured. Without opportunities to express feelings elsewhere, the resulting disempowerment would often burn out to indifference and lethargy. I watched a bright, newly-qualified staff nurse slowly sink under just such circumstances. A lot of the responsibility for this has to be with management teams who fail to prioritise the dissemination of information to the 'shop floor' or don't engage in open consultation but blindly impose short-term money-saving strategies by, for example, limiting the amount of time for shift overlap. In the nine months I was on one particular ward handover time was cut from half an hour to ten minutes for a ward of 25 people. With such restricted time how can you expect accurate information to be passed on to those working closely together let alone more distant professionals – the ripple effect is a given. Lapses in care and 'accidents' are inevitable consequences and must increase time and money spent investigating incidents and resolving complaints.

Apart from the ever-increasing pressure of working within a system of limited resources, constantly changing beliefs, policies and procedures, and a mix of professionals with different understandings, there's also the inevitable imbalances in power that exist in any hierarchical situation. The understandable insecurities, jealousies and rivalry that go alongside provide more than adequate ingredients for communication breakdown. Different professionals will form different opinions according to their background and the quality and quantity of time spent with the individual involved. Often those with most contact are the least involved in decisions made about care. So, for example, health care assistants may have no voice. With limited time and opportunity for all-inclusive discussions, reaching a consensus of opinion is rare. Consequently those with most influence and authority usually make the decisions. As a result there is the potential for those in disagreement, or left out of the process, to feel undermined – that their judgement and viewpoint is redundant or not valued. In addition decisions may go unexplained to those carrying them out. Sometimes this leaves the way open for dissent. I asked one nurse why he would not follow my care plan. In his answer he made no secret of his contempt for the consultant, said he disagreed with my diagnosis and care plan and went on to give his reasons for a different formulation. It was sad that his relationship with the consultant was such that he was unable to have the conversation with him instead of me.

Written reports are often relied on as the most usual way for professionals and agencies to keep in touch with each other. They have the advantage of being available to all (including patient/client) – and seem to be transparent. However the method may give rise to duplicity, staff recording one thing and saying another – particularly given the sensitivity of 'patient access'. Relying on written records alone can mean there is less emphasis on discussion and so misinterpretations and errors go unquestioned. Records are also a static representation in a fluid process and so soon lose their validity and yet at the same time can crystallise our view of an individual (as in my example at the beginning). It may be hard to move on from (or question) initial formulations and the labelling that subsequently occurs.

It's an unfortunate reality that we seldom notice the vehicle unless there's malfunction – smooth operations go unnoticed in silence. In view of this it would be remiss to ignore here the majority of my experience in favour of the hiccups. In general I was fortunate enough to receive skilled and professional help from people who communicated well with each other. In particular the consultant psychiatrist, psychologist, specialist nurse and community keyworker complemented each other well, generally functioning cohesively to enable others to understand the philosophy of care. They provided a secure and consistent foundation.

So what helped them function so well together?

Certainly there was the potential for problems – all were from different professional backgrounds (some from different cultures), with different levels of responsibility, serving different geographical areas, some lived under constant threat of closure and job insecurity. But what I observed was this: I saw commitment to and respect for individuality and difference; interactions that were transparent and honest; an awareness of shared responsibility; the flexibility to embrace and adapt to new ideas; role confidence with recognition of the boundaries; realistic expectations of working within the constraints of an inadequate system – an ability to use its strengths and accept its limitations; and well-established systems for networking.

Humans are, by nature, complex animals. Communicating within and between groups of individuals, those complexities may be seen as complications. Developing channels of communication that are enabling requires open reflection of the issues, courage to challenge inertia and a willingness and commitment to change.

SIXTY

AN OBJECT LESSON

Cicely Herbert

I'm to be an exhibit
in the lecture theatre today
important consultants are gathered there
to hear what others say.

I have to display my mended leg
held rigid with metal rods
to a roomful of medical men
bone-setters and orthopods.
   So wheel me, porter, wheel me
   in my supermarket trolley
   out of this humdrum ward.
It's ages before they can see me
they're studying X-rays and charts
and I must sit in the subway
before my performance starts.

Now the doors are opened
they're beckoning me inside
when I'm facing rows of men in suits
I'm shy and there's nowhere to hide.
   Oh, wheel me, porter, wheel me
   in my supermarket trolley
   far from their expert eye.

Source: Herbert, C, Henley, WE. *In Hospital*. London: KATABASIS, 1992.
Reproduced by permission.

My handsome doctor's become quite distant
he's pointing at me with a stick
when he asks for relevant questions
there's a silence and I feel sick.

Then someone says something in Latin
and asks if I can move it.
He regrets that I can't yet retract my foot
and I can't, though I try to disprove it.
    Oh, wheel me, porter, wheel me
    in my supermarket trolley
    to the warmth of Ward 2/2.
When the demonstration is over
and I can go back to bed
I feel that I've failed an important exam.
Was there something I should have said?

INDEX